HOW NOT TO LOOK OLD

CHARLA KRUPP

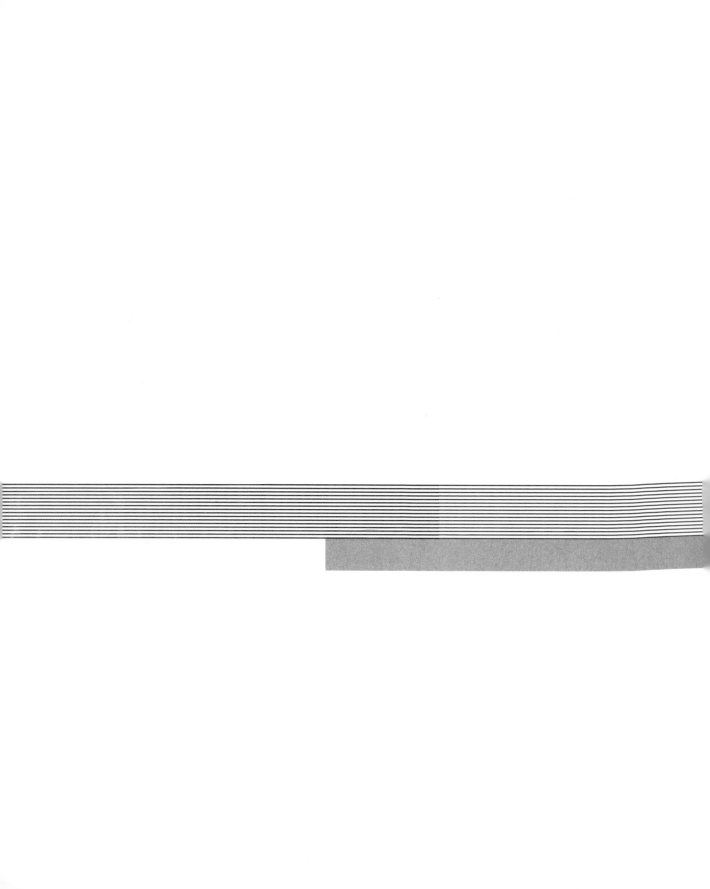

HOW NOT TO LOOK OLD

FAST AND EFFORTLESS WAYS TO LOOK

10 Years Younger
10 Pounds Lighter
10 Times Better

CHARLA KRUPP

Developed and Written with The Stonesong Press

SPRINGBOARD PRESS

NEW YORK   BOSTON

Springboard Press
Hachette Book Group USA
237 Park Avenue, New York, NY 10017
Visit our Web site at
www.HachetteBookGroupUSA.com

First Edition: January 2008

Springboard Press is an imprint of
Grand Central Publishing. The Springboard name and logo is a trademark of
Hachette Book Group USA, Inc.
How Not to Look Old™ is a trademark of Charla Krupp.

Author's Note: This book includes the author's opinions based on her research and experience. The author believes that the information in this book is accurate as of August 1, 2007. The author and the publisher are not affiliated with the companies whose products or services are referred to in this book, do not endorse or sponsor any such products or services, and are not responsible for any such products or services. The information in this book is not intended to be a substitute for medical and other professional advice; you are advised to consult with your health care professional with regard to matters that may require diagnosis or medical attention.

Library of Congress Cataloging-in-Publication Data
Krupp, Charla.
    How not to look old: fast and effortless ways to look 10 years younger, 10 pounds lighter, 10 times better / Charla Krupp. — 1st ed.
        p.   cm.

    Summary: "Boot camp for a younger, hipper makeover, packed with no-holds-barred advice on little beauty and fashion changes that pay off big time."
— Provided by the publisher.
    ISBN-13: 978-0-446-58114-1
    ISBN-10: 0-446-58114-3
    1. Middle-aged women — Psychology.   2. Middle-aged women — Attitudes.   3. Middle-aged women — Physiological aspects.   4. Beauty, Personal.   5. Feminine beauty (Aesthetics)
6. Women — Psychology.   7. Self-esteem in women.   8. Body image in women.   I. Title.
HQ1059.4K78   2008
646.7'042 — dc22   2007016654

10   9   8   7   6   5   4   3   2   1

IMAGO

Design by Cicero deGuzman Jr.

Developed and Written with The Stonesong Press

Printed in the United States of America

Dedicated to
(in order of appearance):

My mom, Terry Krupp, my first beauty and style guru.
My mentor, Ruth Whitney, the late great editor in chief of *Glamour,* who knew I was a beauty editor
before I did.
My husband, Richard Zoglin, who never complained about a dining table constantly covered
in cosmetics and who found time to help with my book while writing his own!

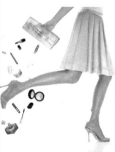

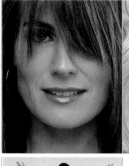
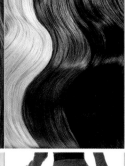
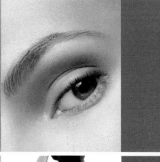

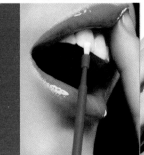
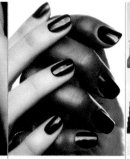
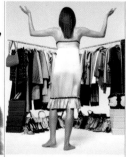
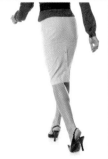
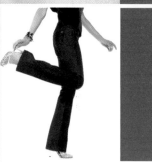

CONTENTS

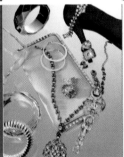
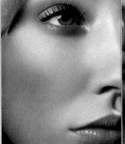
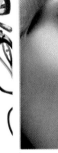
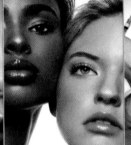
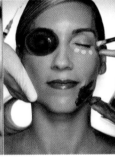
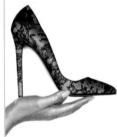
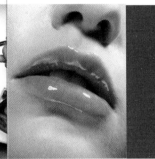
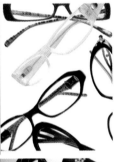
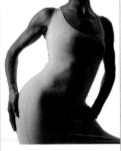
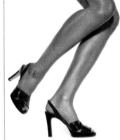
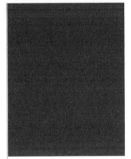

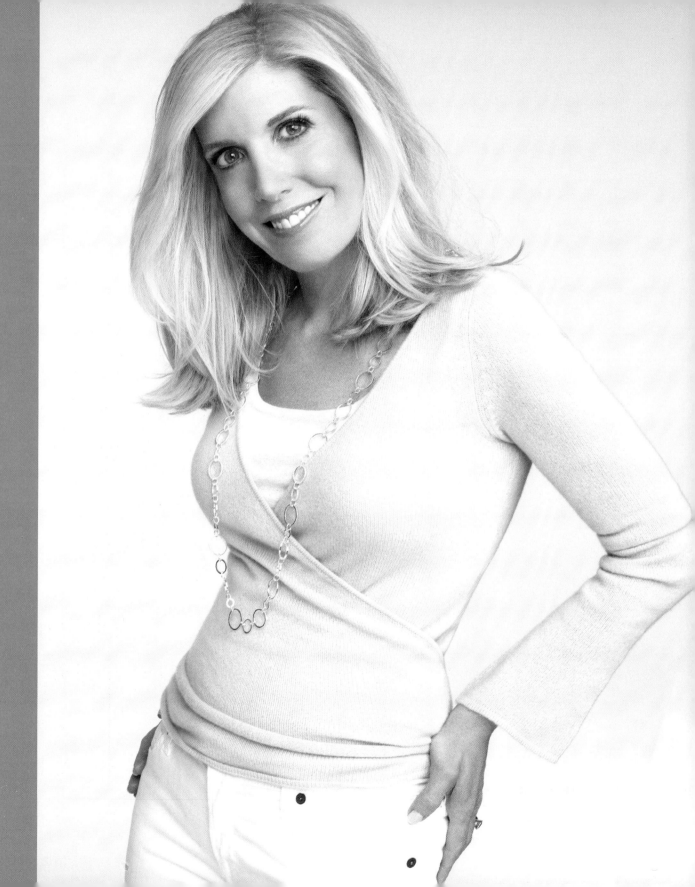

FORGET
AGING GRACEFULLY

All right, I'm just going to come out and say it. **Aging sucks.** As my generation of women hits forty, fifty, sixty, we are for the first time discovering things about our faces and bodies that we never noticed before. Icky things such as age spots, crow's-feet, gray hair, chin hair, marionette lines, saggy boobs, spider veins, bunions — need I go on? I don't think so. You know what I'm talking about. The question is, *What are you — what are we — going to do about it?*

We're going to fight aging — and we're going to look great doing it.

Whether it's by our sheer numbers (seventy-eight million strong — the largest demographic group in history) or our sheer chutzpah, we baby boomers are pros at shaking things up as we hit each decade. We know how to do this. From rock music in the sixties, to "Me Generation" therapy in the seventies, to the "Let's Get Physical" fitness boom of the eighties, to the spa fad of the nineties, to the green movement of today, our generation has no problem rewriting the rules to suit our needs as we move past life's milestones. Now that we are going to live to be a hundred, our mission is to reinvent retirement and the golden years. Although we haven't nailed that yet (for some of us, retirement is still a ways away), we already know that we're not going to just stand there like a bunch of Willy Lomans and accept our gold watch with a thank-you and a smile at the retirement party (if we even get the watch — or the party). Neither are we likely to be sailing into the sunset spending our retirement playing golf or tennis, or sitting around the pool with a cocktail in hand. **What else aren't we going to do?**

Younger and hipper is a concept I'll use a lot, so let's just say Y&H from now on. As opposed to looking like an old lady (OL for short). The chapters in this book are organized from head to toe, from "Cut Some Bangs" to "Step into Sexy Heels." This master list of to-dos leads to even more things you can do to get gorgeous. If you go chapter by chapter and cross off the to-dos as you go, you will look ten years younger, ten pounds lighter, and ten times better. Maybe even *more* than ten years younger. At the start of each chapter, you'll find the words "Look *X* Years Younger," which show the approximate number of years this to-do will set back the clock. Don't add all these up, or you'll be back in the womb! Instead, use the number to gauge the visual impact you'll get from doing this to-do.

Ever wonder why some fifty-year-olds look like they're forty and others look like they're sixty? Today everyone wants to look ten years younger than they are. Forty is the new thirty, fifty is the new forty, and so on. Looking younger is not all about lucky genes. It takes work. But if you do too much

■ We're not going to grow old gracefully (or gratefully).

■ We're not going to celebrate our wrinkles (you've got to be kidding).

The last bullet point on page 3 is where this book comes in. *How Not to Look Old* is the boomer manifesto: a comprehensive plan of attack on aging, all those little beauty and style tweaks that you can (and should!) do to look younger and hipper — and still show up for work the next day.

work, the comments you'll be hearing will not be, "Wow! You look fabulous!" but rather, "*Wow! What did you do?*"

This book is not about extreme makeovers. I have nothing against plastic surgery. In fact, I have personal experience to share (see chapter 6). But I don't think plastic surgery guarantees that you're going to look young. You might not have any wrinkles after a face-lift, but if you look like you had work done, you're obviously old enough to have a face-lift! So who are you fooling? A face frozen in time is the face of a Woman Who Has Had Too Much Work Done. As fashion designer Isaac Mizrahi recently said to me, "I think plastic surgery is the most aging thing in the world. If you want to look seventy, boy, get a face-lift. Get your lips done."

Another reason why there's no chapter on plastic surgery is that many of us just don't have time for downtime. Instant gratification is part of our DNA. We want fast fixes. That's why there's also no mention of the fact that diet and exercise are essential to looking younger and staying healthy over the long haul. There isn't a woman alive who doesn't already know that. Eating salmon and doing yoga are good things to do for sure, but they won't give you the instant results that the to-dos in this book will. We want results. Real results. Visible results. Other antiaging books tell you to run a bath, light a candle, chant and practice acceptance. Not this one. I've tried all that — and guess what? It doesn't work!

called on my friends — some of the best beauty and fashion pros in the biz — to share their secrets throughout this book. Not ridiculous, over-the-top ideas, but advice we all can put to use. I know they are the real deal — many of them have worked their magic on me. And even though most live in New York City, as I do, their suggestions apply to all types of women, and encompass all price points.

At this stage, we don't take kindly to spending $350 or even $35 on a wrinkle cream and then finding out six to eight weeks later that those little lines bleeding off the top of your lips have not disappeared. In my former years, I was beauty director at *Glamour* and editor in chief of the late beauty Web site eve.com, and I've made a career out of being a beauty guinea pig. There's nothing I won't put on my face in the name of beauty. Magazines are packed with advertisers' products, and we're inundated with commercials and ads, but how do we know what really works? At the end of most chapters, you'll find my Brilliant Buys,

■ We're not going to join the Women Who Have Had Too Much Work Done club (like our mothers and their friends).

■ We're not going to look old.

What works is going to the dermatologist and, if necessary, making her or him your new best friend. From Botox to fillers to peels to lasers, there are so many noninvasive options in our beauty arsenal these days. To find what works best, I've

the results of my heavy lifting. I personally tested more than one thousand beauty products, most of which had already landed on "best of beauty" lists in the major magazines. I am a very tough customer. To make the cut, my Brilliant Buys had to (1) deliver results, (2) be user-friendly, (3) look good enough to keep on the bathroom shelf, and (4) not be insanely expensive. Somewhere along the line, we learned that the more money we spend, the

Looking younger will keep you in the game longer when everyone around you is a kid.

better the results will be. I'm here to tell you that that is simply not true. Some of the best cleansers, moisturizers, mascaras, foundations, and shampoos can be found at Target.

The older you get, the more you need maintenance. This book is very much about maintenance; in fact, many of the to-dos are offered in a high-, medium-, or low-maintenance menu. In Nora Ephron's hilarious book *I Feel Bad About My Neck,* she says this about maintenance: "Maintenance takes up so much of my life that I barely have time to sit down at the computer. You know what maintenance is, I'm sure. Maintenance is what they mean when they say, 'After a certain point it's just patch patch patch.'" The daily, weekly, and monthly patch, patch, patch is the difference between a fifty-year-old who looks forty and a fifty-year-old who looks sixty. The truth is, **we cannot afford to let ourselves go!**

For our generation, looking younger isn't just about vanity. (Well, okay, sometimes we *are* a little vain.) Looking good is about our personal and financial survival. We are the first generation of women in which the majority of us went to college and then to work. But many of us do not have husbands (rich or otherwise) to support us. Many of us do not have kids to take care of us, or kids who *want* to take care of us. Many of us are on our own, and *we need to stay in the workplace until we say it's time to go.*

And let's not fool ourselves: looking good is

key to keeping our jobs. Studies on attractiveness have shown that people who are better-looking, younger, and slimmer are more likely to get a job and keep it — as well as to win friends, influence people, and keep their partners interested. In psychologist Ellen Berscheid's studies of the 1970s and 1980s, *Overview of the Psychological Effects of Physical Attractiveness,* she concludes that people believe "what is beautiful, is good." That is, we attribute positive qualities such as kindness, sincerity, and warmth to people who are good-looking and negative qualities to people who are not. Alex Kuczynski, in her book *Beauty Junkies,* analyzes a number of attractiveness studies and concludes, "To get a good job in the United States, the scientific data suggests you not only have to be relatively trim and good-looking but you have to be young."

Looking younger will keep you in the game longer when everyone around you is a kid. It's a no-brainer. Many of us have had the experience of being at work and realizing that we are the oldest person around the conference table — and not by a few years. We've reached the age where some of our colleagues are young enough to be our kids. We have to look younger to help level the playing field.

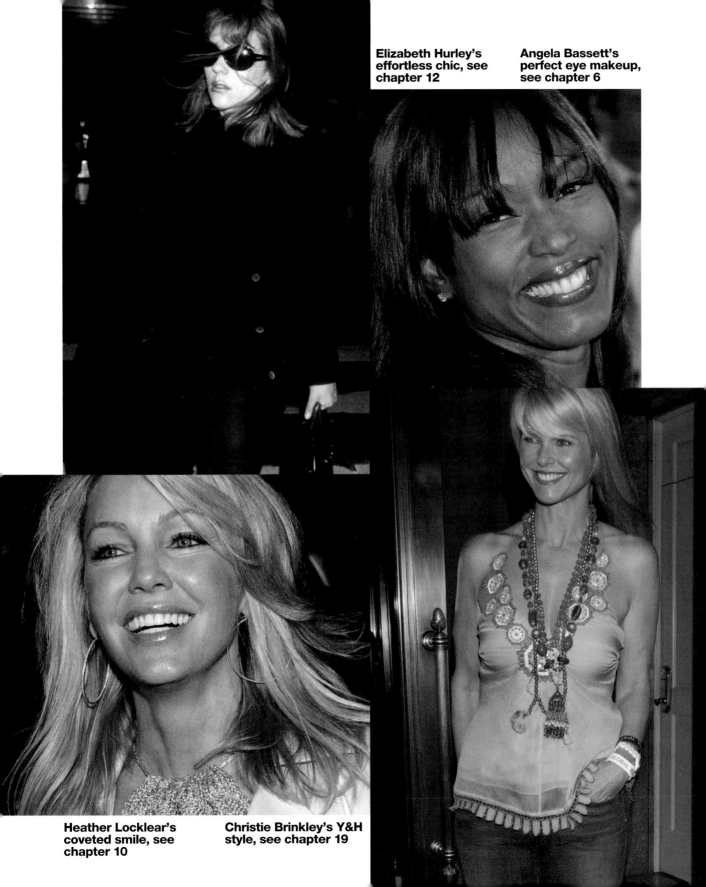

Elizabeth Hurley's effortless chic, see chapter 12

Angela Bassett's perfect eye makeup, see chapter 6

Heather Locklear's coveted smile, see chapter 10

Christie Brinkley's Y&H style, see chapter 19

But shouldn't we be showing off our wrinkles? Shouldn't we be proud to go gray? Yes, that would be awesome in an ideal world. But that's not the way the world is today. Only when women who look as "good" as Morley Safer and Andy Rooney are allowed to thrive well into their seventies and even eighties on the public stage will it be safe for us to let ourselves go without endangering our livelihoods and our legacies. Until then, to keep our paychecks and our self-esteem, we need to look young; we need to look current. And the stakes have been raised so high that we need to look *fabulous.*

Make no mistake: this doesn't mean you need to look twenty. You need to look youthful, as if you're still swimming in the stream of all things current. You're going to look out of it if you show up in a fussy suit when everyone else at the office is in jeans. You're going to look OL if you have a "helmet head" loaded with hair spray when everyone else has long, lush locks. So how do you look current without wearing a miniskirt, flip-flops, and an iPod plugged into your ear?

How Not to Look Old is about looking young without looking ridiculous. Unapologetically written for the over-forty generation, this is a cheat sheet that cuts through the clutter of what's in, what's hot, what you must have this season — in other words, what you are presented with when you pick up most fashion magazines, which are nearly all targeted to the eighteen- to thirty-five-year-old set. The problem is that what looks good on Scarlett or Lindsay or Paris will probably not look good on you. And even though I spent my career as an editor working in the trenches of fashion magazines, I am not, by any means, a fashionista. In fact, I am the one who sits in on the fashion run-throughs and says about the bag that costs $7,500, "Do you know anyone who's going to buy that?" I grew up in Wilmette, Illinois, and

my husband is from Kansas City, Missouri. We go back to both places a lot. I know that what plays in New York and LA will not necessarily translate. We're bombarded with inappropriate fashions, and it's not just from magazines. As I'm writing, I'm watching a morning TV style segment showing crotch-high minidresses and short-short suits for spring. Hello? What about us? Is there anything that we might put on without looking ridiculous? Part of the mission of this book is to reinvigorate the term "age appropriate." Every single beauty and style tip is presented with that in mind. Look at the photos, and you'll know exactly what's too young/too old/just right.

Despite all our good intentions, there are little things we all do that can betray our best efforts and scream OL to the outside world. Right now, for instance, are you

■ **in dark lipstick?**

■ **wearing an eyeglass chain around your neck?**

■ **covering your face with a mask of foundation?**

■ **wearing granny pants or mommy jeans?**

■ **wearing a bra that doesn't boost the girls up halfway between your shoulders and your elbows?**

From now on, you'll be on high alert to the telltale signs that can creep up on you and threaten your look if you're not paying attention. Each chapter starts with a "shout out" called "Nothing Ages You Like . . ." covering things such as:

- **Too-long hair that's parted down the middle**

- **A solid block of hair color**

- **Gray or white brow hairs**

- **Half-glasses**

- **Obvious lip liner**

- **Yellow teeth**

- **Dragon-lady nails**

The point is, if you've been outlining your lips the same way since college, you're overdue for a change. And throughout this book, you'll find "The Newer Way to . . ." do everything to make yourself look modern, not stale.

Before many of us can climb out of our beauty and fashion ruts, we need to escape our comfort zones. And to do that successfully, we need a new mind-set. Think, "*You,* only in a gorgeous new dress." We're not talking inner beauty here. We're paying attention only to your outer beauty, the package you present to the world. Think this is superficial? Sorry, but this is the real world. Every day, people size you up in a nanosecond, making judgments that could affect your future based on whether your nails are too long or your skirt is too short. You can't afford not to look your best every time you step out the front door.

You know that the benefits of looking younger and better are not superficial at all. I hate to use

this word, because it is so overused, but it is *empowering* to pass a mirror and think, "Wow, I look great!" It gives you a lift. Every time I walk out of the hair salon blown-out and blonder, I feel as if I could conquer the world. Our looks and our self-esteem are inextricably wired. You need to invest time, money, and interest in *you,* because if you don't *look good,* you don't *feel good* about yourself. And if you don't look and feel good on a daily basis, no one close to you is going to feel good either. If you have any doubts about the "look good, feel better" connection, volunteer at a women's organization such as Bottomless Closet or Dress for Success and see how a new outfit can make a down-and-out woman suddenly feel optimistic and hopeful about her future.

How Not to Look Old is about looking Y&H, but to truly be Y&H, you need to embrace a youthful attitude. You need to jump into life and wrap your arms around change. Whether it's beauty or fashion or life in general, what is truly OL? Being too invested in the status quo. I hate it when people say, "That's not the way it's done." So? Are you saying that you can't ever change the way it's done? Why not? Only OL people make a big deal about change. That's not going to be you!

What's great about coming of age at this particular point in time is that unlike our mothers, we have so many things we can do to look Y&H before resorting to extreme measures and joining the Women Who Have Had Too Much Work Done club. What follows is the to-do list to end all to-do lists. **Here's to looking younger, feeling better, and winning the battle.** If I can do it, so can you.

1

ARE YOU
HIGH, MEDIUM, OR LOW
MAINTENANCE?

've been fascinated by maintenance ever since I learned there was a word to describe all those little things women do to make themselves look better and feel better on an ongoing basis. I love to know what other women do, where they go, how much time and money they're willing to shell out. When I consider the women I know, our maintenance levels run the gamut depending on where we live and what we do. My sister-in-law Janet and I laugh about how two women in the same family can be so polar opposite. When she was traveling through Africa on the back of a date truck, all she needed was toothpaste, a toothbrush, and toilet paper. Now that she's home, her beauty needs don't extend beyond a moisturizing mist from the health food store. I, on the other hand, could open up a store with the beauty products I have collected over the years. (The scary thing was, when I set out to test-drive all the products for the Brilliant Buys you'll find in these chapters, I discovered at least half of them in my house.)

Surely, some women are so obsessed with beauty and style that maintenance is a full-time job. Whenever you tell them about a new procedure,

they've already booked the appointment. Whenever you tell them about the latest must-have, they're already on the waiting list. Then there are the bare-basics women (granted, Janet is the extreme) who can't be bothered with any of that fuss.

Just knowing all the options that are available — even if you don't have the time, desire, or cash to partake — helps democratize the injustice of beauty. If you didn't luck out in the gene pool, it's comforting to know that you can always buy flawless skin, gorgeous hair, and a big, white, flashy smile. At *Glamour,* we once interviewed the comedian Sandra Bernhard and asked her if she'd rather be smart, pretty, or rich. "Smart, then rich," she answered. "You can always buy pretty!"

I'm all for full disclosure about the heavy lifting some women do because it's healthy for our collective self-esteem. When modern-day goddesses walk the red carpet, we now know that it took a village — and the dedication of an Olympic athlete in training. That's progress, because years ago no one in Hollywood would admit to having any help at all. I remember writing a *Glamour* feature titled "The Best Beauty Decision I Ever Made," and I practically had to get to the Zs in my Rolodex before find-

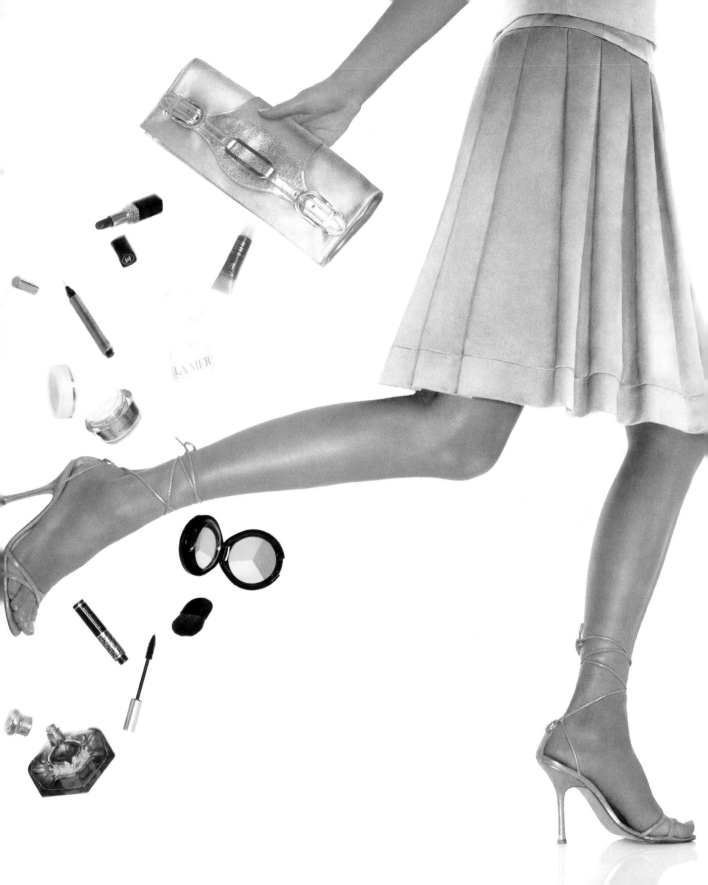

ing enough actresses who would share anything beyond "I drink a lot of water." Gee, thanks! Today the veil has been lifted, and many stars graciously acknowledge the efforts of their style squad: "I'd like to thank my hairdresser, my skin doctor . . ." And when they go on the record about having a bit of Botox, well, even that small injection of truth about their red-carpet dermatology prep is better than pretending they just rolled out of bed looking awards-show ready.

A FUNNY THING HAPPENED ON THE WAY TO THE SALON

I may never have ended up as a beauty director — which has now led to writing this book — if it weren't for my fascination with maintenance. Back in the nineties, I was the entertainment editor for *Glamour* magazine. But I wrote an article about beauty that defined high, medium, and low maintenance and gave examples of women who embraced each category. I was the high-maintenance poster girl — complete with a photo of me having my hair cut and my fingers and toes tended to simultaneously. My annual upkeep at the time cost $7,398. It was a thrill to give my longtime beauty team the credit they deserved and also to get a taste of what other women do and eschew.

Years later, when I was working at *In Style*, Ruth Whitney, *Glamour*'s longtime editor in chief, called me and offered me the job of beauty director. "I don't know anything about beauty!" I said to her. "But," she argued, "you wrote the best beauty piece the magazine ever ran." The rest, as they say, is herstory.

Thankfully, most of us don't have paparazzi anxiously waiting to capture our slightest fashion or beauty misstep. But we all have our tipping points when it comes to maintenance. Do too much, and you might feel bad about having been talked into a $200 jar of moisturizer or joining the growing ranks of Women Who Have Had Too Much Work Done. By this stage in your life, you know your own tipping point — you're the expert on you. You know when you've gone too far — or when you look like hell because you're not treating yourself well.

Defining your maintenance level is all about defining your priorities: who you are and what you aspire to be. There are things I *wish* I could do. Like when I heard that *Vogue* editor in chief Anna Wintour had a hairdresser and makeup artist come to her house every morning. I would *love* that — although I wouldn't love to pay for it. These days, when everyone is on overload 24/7, maintenance is as much about time as it is about the ease with which you can wipe away your credit card balance. As I write this, I'm glad you can't see my nails. I don't have twenty minutes to run across the street and get a manicure, nor do I have time to do it myself. And then there are some beauty routines you never, ever have time for. These fall into the "life's too short" category. Mine include waiting for moisturizer to dry after showering, massaging in cellulite cream every day for six weeks in the hope of seeing improvement, and at-home paraffin kits for hands. (I've had one sitting unopened in my bathroom since the year 2000.) I love regular pedicures, but I'd brave snowy streets in flip-flops before I'd sit in a salon till my toes dried.

We all have our unwritten "life's too short" lists, our wish lists, and our "absolutely, no matter what happens, can't live without this" lists. Take this quiz to determine whether you're currently a high-, medium-, or low-maintenance woman (and what that really means).

Define Your Maintenance Level
TAKE THIS QUIZ TO FIND OUT WHERE YOU ARE.

1. You never leave the house without

a. a full face of makeup.

b. some lipstick and mascara.

c. a clean face.

2. Your closet

a. should be photographed for a magazine.

b. is due for its seasonal clean-out.

c. still holds your cat suit.

3. When you're traveling, you wear

a. business attire.

b. pants and a nice sweater.

c. whatever is comfiest.

4. On a rare day off, you

a. schedule an appointment with your dermatologist, hair colorist, manicurist, or personal shopper.

b. meet a friend at the mall.

c. sleep.

5. You won the lottery and must spend the jackpot only on yourself. You

a. get a face-lift.

b. shop for a whole new wardrobe.

c. buy a new car.

6. If you could be locked in a store all night, you would want it to be

a. Neiman Marcus.

b. Sephora.

c. Williams-Sonoma.

7. You received a gift certificate to a day spa. You

a. immediately book a massage, facial, or something else on the spa menu.

b. eventually get around to making an appointment.

c. let it expire or regift it.

8. If you can't read the tiny type on the back of the tube of self-tanner, you

a. slip on a pair of cool readers.

b. grab your drugstore readers.

c. squint and hope for the best.

9. You wash your face with

a. whatever your dermatologist prescribes.

b. a prestige brand cleanser.

c. whatever's in the soap dish.

10. You received a last-minute invite to a dressy cocktail party. You

a. wear the new dress hanging in your closet.

b. make do with your standby black skirt and sparkly sweater.

c. don't go because you have nothing to wear and no time to shop.

11. If you had a party, would your hair colorist and hairstylist be invited?

a. Of course, they're friends.

b. Yes, but they're the same person.

c. What colorist?

12. Your handbag that you tote day in, day out

a. is one of several must-have bags of the moment.

b. is the one new bag you buy every season.

c. is the same one you've used for years.

13. Your crow's-feet

a. are gone.

b. are a constant source of worry.

c. never cross your mind.

Turn this page to see how you rate.

ARE YOU HIGH, MEDIUM, OR LOW MAINTENANCE?

STAR STYLES
The Older They Get, the Better They Look

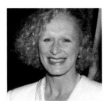

**Glenn Close
in 1995 . . .**

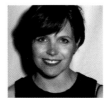

**Katie Couric
in 1996 . . .**

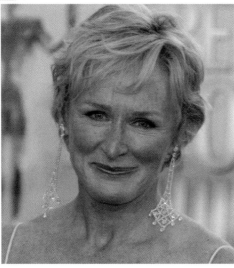

In 2005

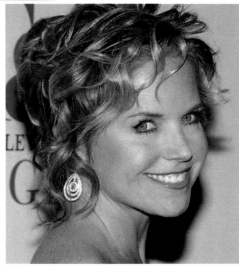

In 2006

ARE YOU HIGH, MEDIUM, OR LOW MAINTENANCE?

Obviously, the "a" answers are high maintenance, the "b's" medium, and the "c's" low. If you're like most women, your answers are a mix of all three letters. I think we all know the following stereotypes.

HIGH: You're doing every single thing you know to look great — whatever the time, whatever the cost. And chances are you're always hearing how fantastic you look. The downside here (if there is a downside) is that (1) it's exhausting, (2) it's expensive, and (3) there is definitely a point of no return. Just keep in mind that Women Who Have Had Too Much Work Done can look OL. Being high maintenance is one thing; looking it is another. You could be in danger of trying too hard. To look Y&H, you might find that sometimes less equals more.

MEDIUM: You aspire to look as great as someone who is high maintenance, but you can't imagine devoting that many hours and burning through that much cash. You're more likely to cherry-pick, spending time and money on things that give you the most bang for your buck. You feel good about yourself and confident about your choices, but you might want to give in and go for

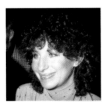

**Barbra Streisand
in 1980 . . .**

In 2004

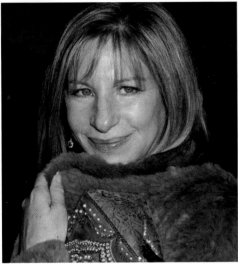

**Bette Midler
in 1987 . . .**

In 2004

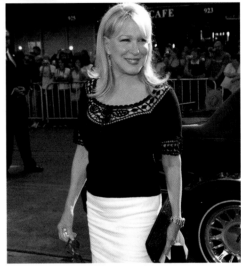

the "wow!" occasionally, rather than settling for the "good enough."

LOW: You don't invest a lot of time and money in yourself because it hasn't been a big priority in your life. But now you're at the point where you look in the mirror and ask, "What else can I do?" Have *you* come to the right place! On the pages ahead, you'll find plenty of ways to ramp up. For starters, stop feeling guilty. Guilt is so OL!

But no one is a pure stereotype; we're always mixing our maintenance options, trading up and

trading down, spending our time and money where we need it and where it feels right. Welcome to the way in which real women live! What lies ahead in this book are the most current menus detailing all your high-, medium-, and low-maintenance options for freshening up everything from your hair color to your toenail polish, your eyewear to your bras. Whip through these chapters, and you're on your way to becoming even more of a mix master. Think of yourself as a work in progress; you always want to be evolving. And FYI, this work is never done! I'm not going to lie to you; it *is* work, but it's fun work. And the results are so worth it. Why *not* be one of those women who keeps getting better- and better-looking? These stars did it, and now you will, too.

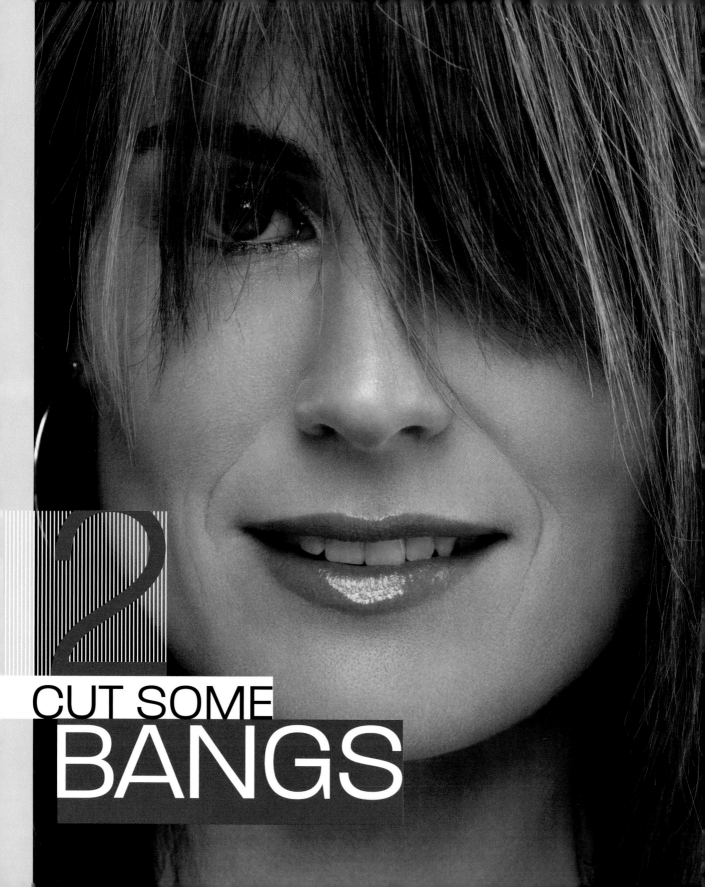

2
CUT SOME
BANGS

NOTHING AGES YOU LIKE...
TOO-SHORT BANGS... TOO-LONG HAIR PARTED DOWN THE MIDDLE... HELMET HEAD... HIGH HAIR... AN UPDO... VISIBLY THINNING HAIR

For my mother's birthday, I decided to frame a collage of family photographs. Sift through hundreds of pictures culled from the decades, and you, too, may uncover an enlightening hairstyle retrospective. Yes, I found photos with criminally bad haircuts that I wanted to rip up. But the process was incredibly valuable, because there was one constant in all the good haircuts, and it was — you guessed it — bangs. After discussing this aha moment with Chris Cusano, who cuts my hair at the Red Door Spa at Elizabeth Arden NYC, he confirmed that once you reach a certain age, you look better with bangs. Almost everybody does.

Bangs are a cheap and easy way to chic up your look. They also accentuate the positive and camouflage the negative (a common theme that cuts across many categories). This haircut cure-all hides a large forehead, a wrinkled forehead, or a receding hairline. At the same time, a soft fringe of hair falling along the side of your face draws attention up to your eyes (which should still be sparkling) and deflects scrutiny from your jaw (which may be a little slack or saggy).

HOW TO GET A BANG-UP JOB
So you're going to go to your hairstylist and get banged — unless your hair is too curly or textured or you have a stubborn cowlick. In those cases, bangs aren't going to work. They'll pouf out, and the fight to keep them flat is not worth fighting.

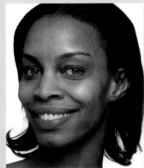 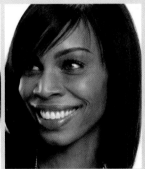

TOO OLD: Jillian with no bangs

JUST RIGHT: she cut back the years with a quick snip.

For everyone else, don't settle on any old bangs. There are Y&H bangs and OL bangs. To get the desired face-framing fringe, your best bets are bangs that are long, thick, and straight or side-swept, angled, or graduated. Anything too severe or geometric will be hard-edged and unflattering, such as those really short bangs that end halfway up your forehead. I know a few super-stylish women who can pull this off and look iconic, but bangs that short make most of us look vintage, dowdy, or, worse, OL.

No matter what the magazines claim is the must-have cut of the moment, stick to your bangs — or some variation. Bangs have their hot seasons, but they're never really out of style. Get a trim at least every three or four months when you see your hairdresser. Resist the urge to snip them yourself in between visits; it's best to leave the scissors in the hands of a pro.

CHANGE IS ALWAYS IN THE HAIR

Once you reach a certain age, you've probably had every hairstyle imaginable and have zeroed in on what's best for you. But even though your days of wild experimentation are over (you're not going to shave your head like Britney Spears), it's still good to keep your style evolving. What does that mean? We're talking subtle changes to keep you from getting stuck in a hair rut. Do you have friends or relatives who haven't changed their hair since high school? I do! That long, straight, flat hair parted down the middle from your teens and twenties will only accentuate your current age if you're still sporting it. Styles change, and so does your face, so try tiny tweaks such as playing with the thickness of your bangs (as long as you don't grow them out altogether). Here are some small changes to discuss with your hairdresser.

■ **Cutting angles and layers.** "Once you get the angles around the face, it opens everything up," says Antoinette Guzzo of Frédéric Fekkai, who styled my hair for TV.

■ **Changing your length a bit,** at least seasonally. Maybe wear your hair longer in the summer than in the winter.

■ **Switching your part.** "Most older women have a side part," says Chris Cusano. "Your profile is different on each side. You might want to accentuate the side of your face you like more by parting your hair on that side." (Avoid a middle part, because if there is anything that is off balance about your face, it will surely be highlighted.)

And if you really *do* want a whole new look, forget trying to match your face shape with a specific style (so OL). Just find yourself an amazing hairstylist.

Is It Time You Switched Stylists?

You need to be thrilled with your hairstylist. Good-hair days are worth the investment. If you find that

STAR STYLES
Better Banged

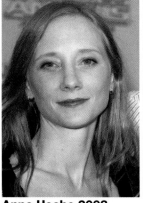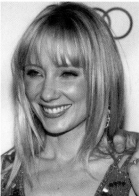

Anne Heche 2003   **2006**

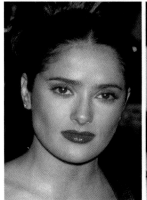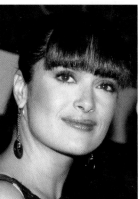

Salma Hayek 1997   **2007**

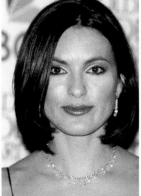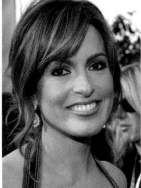

Mariska Hargitay 2000   **2007**

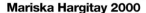

your hairstyle is getting stale and you've run out of ideas to shake it up, it may be time to quit your hairdresser. "If you've been using the same person for a long time, you may have become an exaggerated version of what was once good," says Antoinette Guzzo. "Move on, if someone tells you you can't have a certain style. Everyone can have everything, just a different version of it that's right for your face and your hair and your lifestyle and body shape." And if you find you need to use too many products to look good every day, it's not the right haircut.

You owe it to yourself to sit in a new chair with someone who doesn't know your hair history, who looks at you in a fresh, modern way. In chapter 19, you'll find a list of the best stylists in the country, hopefully in a city near you. I know that breaking up is hard to do, but sometimes you just have to. If you're feeling guilty, you can do the equivalent of what companies do before they fire an employee: give fair warning. Next time you see your stylist, make it crystal clear that you want a younger, fresher look. You can even bring in pages from magazines. If you don't get what you want, your stylist will know why you ended the relationship, especially if you run into each other in the hood and your hair looks more Y&H than ever. You don't have to write a letter; you don't have to call to explain. It's so difficult for some women to put themselves first that they would rather continue with so-so hair than hurt someone's feelings. Don't let this be you! For more ways to find a new stylist (or any beauty pro), read chapter 3.

What If You Can't Find a Style Genius Near You?

Chris Cusano has a client who flies in from London. Antoinette Guzzo has one who hops a plane from Germany. But here's a little nugget that makes me marvel at the ingenuity of modern American women. There are groups of women in Virginia, North Carolina, and Florida who round up their friends and relatives and organize a beauty weekend splitting the cost of flying in a hairdresser from New York. They book the stylist into a hotel, where she spends the weekend cutting the hair of all the women who are in on the deal. "It's actually cheaper than if every woman there were to fly to Manhattan and stay at a hotel," says Antoinette, who has been flown to Cincinnati, Miami, Austin, and St. Croix. High maintenance, yes, but something to keep in the back of your head.

$ Is It Worth It?

The $800 Haircut. In a chic New York City salon, the going rate for a haircut is about $150. But I'm sure you've read about superstar stylists in New York and LA who are charging upwards of $800 for the privilege of laying their hands on your humble head. Do you really need to pay that much to get a great cut? Absolutely not. "It's a haircut," says Chris Cusano. "How much can you do with hair?" Antoinette Guzzo agrees: "It's crazy." If you really want that look, she suggests that you book an appointment at the same salon with someone the Hair God has trained. You'll pay an eighth of the price and get the same look.

YOUR SCALP: A PLACE YOU *CAN* BE TOO THIN

One of the worst things in the What Happens to You When You Get Older file is thinning hair. For some women, it's such an assault to their self-esteem that they can barely talk about it. But don't try to deal with it yourself. As soon as it becomes apparent, talk about it with your doctor. (My dermatologist says that every other woman she sees mentions that her hair is thinning.) Men expect to lose their hair; women do not. But hair loss happens to a whopping 40 percent of menopausal women. Alopecia, as it's called, can occur throughout a woman's life for a variety of reasons: after having a baby, as a reaction to certain medications or illnesses such as cancer, during a time of intense stress, as a result of overprocessing hair or a too-tight hairstyle. In these situations, hair tends to grow back when

Other Hairstyle To-Dos

✔ Keep It Moving

You may be determined to keep every hair in place just the way it was when you left the salon. Warning: hair that doesn't move is so OL. "What looks old is women who are perfectly coiffed, especially when just running around," says Antoinette Guzzo. Worse are women who tease their locks into one high helmet head of hair using too much product. (As they say in country music, the higher the hair, the closer to God.) Y&H hair has bounce. It moves, grooves, gets ruffled, tousled, stirred, and shaken. So lay off the products and insist on a cut that's layered or angled to give you that swing.

✔ Wear It Down

Attending a dressy event and thinking about having your hair swept into a tight updo? Don't. Whether it's a celebrity at an awards show or you at your cousin's wedding, hair pulled tautly on top of the head looks matronly. For one thing, it allows everyone to get a good look at your jaw, your neck, and your collarbone, which you may not want in the line of sight. But even if you have a firm jaw, the more modern way to pull back hair is to make it casual, loose, and a little messy, as if you just pinned it up on your way out the door and couldn't be bothered to catch all the strands. When in doubt, wear your hair down. It's so much sexier.

✔ Grow It (But There Is Such a Thing as Too Long)

Just because you're no longer sixteen doesn't mean you have to pack away your sensuality and chop off your hair. Although a gamine pixie cut can look incredibly sexy,

Teri Hatcher in 1996 . . .

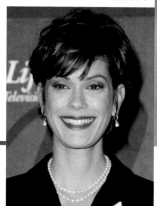

it's not your only option. If your hair is healthy — soft, shiny, no split ends — luxuriate in it, and let others do the same. Long hair is Y&H. There's no point

. . . and in 2006. Short is cute, long is sexier. Grow it!

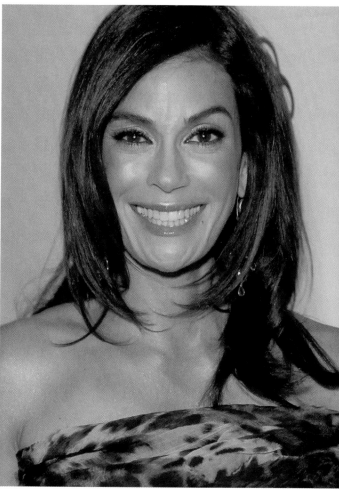

in growing it past the middle of your back, however, as you don't want to look as if you're trying to recapture your teen spirit. A shoulder-grazing cut can look long and lush. When your ends are fried or your hair is starting to thin, it's time to consider chopping off some length.

✔ **Pump Up the Shine**
Young skin glows, as does young hair. So stay away from things that will gunk up the shine. Buckets of hair spray, pomades, and too many styling products can leave your hair looking dull, dull, dull. Counter the damage done with a deep conditioner at least once a week. If your hair is very dry, use it every time you shampoo. Oilier types can get away with less frequent deep conditioning, but for most of us, there's no such thing as overconditioning your hair. PS: Listen to the hair pros when they say that you don't have to wash your hair every single day. It's not good for your hair. Just think of everything you could be doing with all that time!

✔ **Lose the Flakes**
Is there a more instant turnoff than dandruff? Those telltale white flakes on your scalp or clothes are usually the result of dry hair or hair that's been overprocessed. No matter the reason, dandruff sends a message that either you don't care or you haven't walked down the shampoo aisle at the drugstore in years. Getting rid of dandruff is so easy, there's no excuse for it anymore. The formula for Head & Shoulders has improved since the 1960s.

life returns to normal. But for the majority of women who blame menopause, hair loss results from a hormonal shift that is unlikely to correct itself without intervention.

If you notice that your scalp is becoming increasingly visible, your doctor can take a blood test and a scalp analysis to determine why it's happening to you, which will then determine your best course of action. If the cause is not hormonal, some over-the-counter products, such as hair-thickening shampoos and volumizing sprays, might be worth a try. If it is hormonal, your doctor may prescribe Rogaine, which contains minoxidil, the only FDA-approved treatment for hair loss. A 2 percent solution is usually recommended for women (though my derm gives women the same 5 percent solution used for men). Minoxidil is far from perfect — it has to be applied to the entire scalp twice a day, and any regrowth will stop when you stop applying it — but it is worth trying. More likely than helping you grow more hair, it will prevent further loss, so the earlier you start, the better. Just FYI, when you are using minoxidil, watch that it doesn't transfer from your head to your face via your pillow! Dr. Melanie Grossman, a Manhattan dermatologist, told me that facial hair can result from this transfer. (Repeat after me, "Aging sucks.") If minoxidil doesn't work for you, Toppik is an ingenious spray of micro-fiber "hairs" to disguise a bare scalp. And ask your dermatologist about the latest in hair transplants. An increasing number of women are getting them. A hair transplant is neither quick, easy, nor inexpensive, but if it makes you feel good about your hair again, who can put a price on that?

HIGH, MEDIUM, LOW MAINTENANCE . . . THINNING HAIR

HIGH: Why not try extensions? You'd be surprised how many stars wear them. (Unfortunately, this is not a solution for women with male-pattern baldness, but for those who want more volume

TOO YOUNG!

Some things that shouldn't be seen on anyone who has left her twenties:

- A dead-middle part with straight hair, no layers
- High ponytail
- Braids
- Beaded braids
- Thick, structured headbands
- Ribbons
- Kiddie barrettes
- Glitter
- Hair accessories that could be mistaken for toys or charms
- Jaw clips
- Scrunchies

and length.) One of the best (and most expensive) brands is Nylon Integration Hair Extensions from Hairdreams. Made with high-quality human hair, they not only look real and feel great, but they also put far less stress on the hair follicle than most brands. (To find a salon near you, call 310-883-1600 or go to www.hairdreams.com.) This process starts with a preliminary consultation so that your stylist can custom-order extensions that match your hair color and texture. When your extensions arrive, the stylist will attach each one to your existing hair by heating the nylon tip with a special tool until it liquefies. Once this happens, the extension is attached to your natural hair and voila! (Actually, you'll be waiting for the "voila" moment for about four hours, which is how long the process usually takes.) The extensions last for about four months, and during that time, you can swim, shower, and get caught in the rain without worrying that they'll come off. To remove the extensions, you'll have to revisit your stylist so that he or she can unbond them. The process costs $2,500 to $4,000, depending on how many extensions you need.

MEDIUM: Check out synthetic clip-ons. The ones I like best are called HairDo (HSN.com), because you can apply them yourself at home in just a few minutes. If they sound familiar, you might have seen Hollywood hairdresser Ken Paves (who has said he used them on Jessica Simpson) sell them on HSN. They look terrific but last for only one night and won't withstand a heavy downpour (either from your shower or the sky). The good news? The short pieces sell for $85 and the longer ones for $95.

LOW: Make your hair look thicker with just a new cut. Chris Cusano suggests a blunt cut or one that lies flat against the head. "You can't wear something spiky or full; you'll see right through it," he says. "Trying to get your hair full and chopped up in layers doesn't work. To me, it just looks thinner."

THE Y&H MANE GAME FOR WOMEN OF COLOR

Some African American women (like some Caucasian women) may find their hair is not suited to some suggestions in this chapter. For instance, if your hair is too textured, thick, or curly, bangs won't sit well. If you have this type of hair, your first decision is whether you want to wear your hair relaxed or natural (not chemically treated). Salon owner Ellin LaVar (you may know her from her reality TV show, which took place inside her Upper West Side Manhattan salon, Ellin LaVar Hair Designs), who has coiffed Naomi Campbell, Iman, and tennis players Venus and Serena Williams, is a big fan of natural hair because it's ageless. "You can be twenty or sixty, and a natural hairstyle will always work," she says. Let it move as much as possible, and never let it get too big or teased (so OL).

HIGH, MEDIUM, LOW MAINTENANCE HAIR . . . FOR WOMEN OF COLOR

Time vs. Money is Relaxing vs. Weaving. My friend, beauty editor Ayren Jackson-Cannady, who knows more about African American women's hair than I do, thinks that time trumps money here but concedes that it's a close call.

HIGH: Relaxed hair. First, you chemically straighten your hair, then you cut it to, say, shoulder length so that it falls just below the bottom of the ear, with layers framing the face. Relaxed hair requires the most daily upkeep, as it has to be styled with products and hot tools every morning. You also have to get a relaxation touch-up every six weeks, plus visit the salon every other week for a deep-conditioning treatment to strengthen the chemically treated strands — not to mention frequent haircuts. Initial relaxer: $100 to $200; relaxer touch-up: $100; deep conditioning: $30; haircut: $100 or more.

MEDIUM: A weave. A weave may seem pricey, but once you've done it, the upkeep is minimal. To start, your real hair is braided around your head, then extensions are sewn in, cut, and styled. Once you're home, it's wash, condition, and go. Typically, the hair that is woven in is already curly, wavy, or straight, so hot tools don't need to be used. A weave is a lot less compromising to the health of your hair than a relaxer because your real hair is safely tucked away. A weave lasts six to ten weeks and costs about $500.

LOW: Let it go natural. Get a great super-short cut and deep-condition at home. "Natural" in this case does not refer to hair color but to hair texture. If you're going gray, you'll look younger if you color it (see chapter 3).

BRILLIANT BUYS

STYLING FINE HAIR
Bumble and Bumble Thickening Spray, $28.79; cvs.com or bumbleandbumble.com for locations
Fekkai More All-Day Density Styling Whip, $25; Sephora, 877-737-4672 or sephora.com
Phytovolume Actif Volumizing Spray, $28; Sephora, 877-737-4672 or sephora.com

DANDRUFF SHAMPOO
Head & Shoulders Anti-Dandruff Shampoo, $4.99; drugstores and mass retailers

SHAMPOOS
Kérastase Paris Bain Age Recharge, $29; for salons, call 877-748-8357 or kerastase.com
Pantene Pro-V Restoratives Shampoo, $5.75; drugstores and mass retailers

Phytomousse Volume Shampoo, $24, for salons, call 800-55-PHYTO or phyto.com

CONDITIONERS
Garnier Fructis Fortifying Deep Conditioner, $3.99, drug stores and mass retailers
Kérastase Paris Masque Age Recharge, $58, for salons, call 877-748-8357 or kerastase.com

THINNING HAIR
Fekkai More Nighttime Follicle-Boosting Treatment, $35, Sephora, 877-737-4672 or sephora.com
Women's Rogaine Hair Regrowth Treatment, $24.95; Rogaine, 888-835-9712 or rogainedirect.com
NIOXIN System 1 Starter Kit for Fine, Natural, Normal to Thin-Looking Hair, and **NIOXIN** System 5 Starter Kit for Medium, Coarse, Natural, Normal to Thin-Looking Hair, $39.99, 800-628-9890 for locations.

HairMax LaserComb Premium, $545; 866-527-3726 or lasercomb.net
Toppik microfiber hairs, $19.95, toppik.com

HAIR EXTENSIONS
Hairdreams Human Hair Extensions, $800–$3,250; 310-883-1600 or hair-dreams.com for salons
Hair Do, $85 and $95; HSN.com

HAIR TOOLS
T3 Bespoke Labs Evolution Collection Dryer, $300; Sephora, 877-737-4672 or sephora.com; Ulta, ulta.com
CHI Ceramic Flat Iron, $159.95; Farouk, 800-237-9175 or farouk.com
Champion Collection Comb, $6.95; norvabarbersupply.com
Mason Pearson Hair Brushes, $45–$230; Neiman Marcus, 888-888-4757, or whatshebuys.com

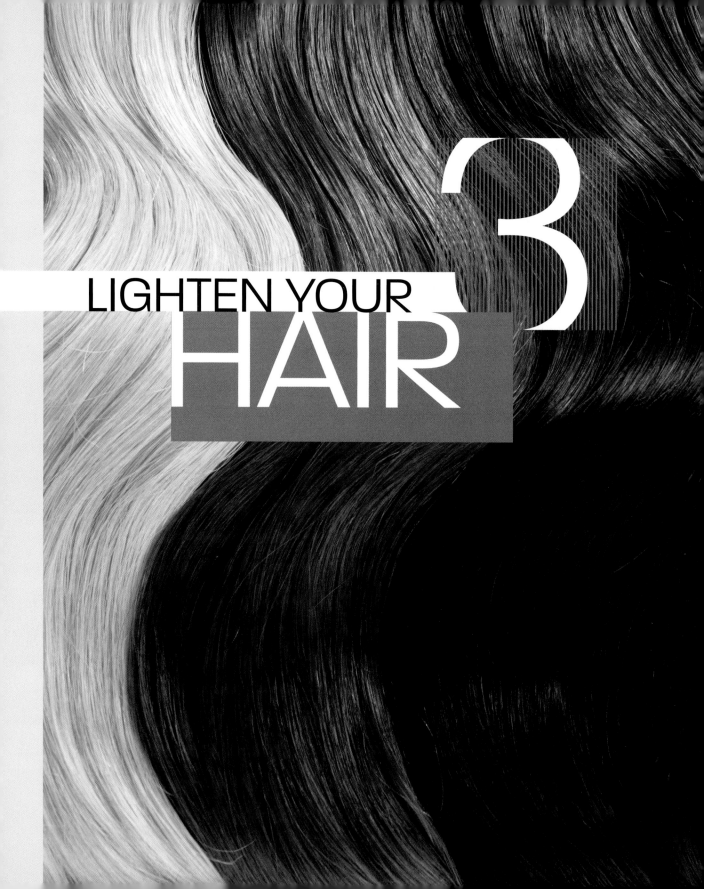

LIGHTEN YOUR HAIR

3

NOTHING AGES YOU LIKE …
TOO-DARK HAIR … A SOLID BLOCK OF HAIR COLOR … DULL HAIR … GRAY HAIR … GRAY ROOTS … ASHY BLOND STREAKS

By this stage in our lives, we all know our best features. Blondness is mine. I started coloring my hair when I was sixteen, when I decided that my boring brunette locks weren't glamorous enough for New Trier West High School. My first colorist was my mother. Armed with a box of Clairol Summer Blonde, we would spend hours together at the bathroom sink, me wearing a rubber cap dotted with holes, she with what looked like a crochet hook to pull the strands through. I've been coloring my hair forever — and love being blond — but lately every other woman I pass on the street is gray. Leave it to the boomer generation to make gray hair hip! I happen to love the look of a sexy silver mane (think Julie Christie in *Away from Her*). But before you join the sisterhood of silver foxes, know that although platinum hair can look cool, it will never look young. Truthfully, it adds ten years. Most of us are only too happy to wash that gray right out of our hair.

I learned the general rule about birthdays and hair color from Brad Johns, global color director at Clairol and national color director of the Red Door Spa at Elizabeth Arden NYC, who has been directing my blondification for more than twenty years: *The older you get, the lighter you go.* This does not mean that every woman should suddenly become a blonde. Not everyone looks better as a blonde, but almost everyone looks better with lightness around her face. Whatever your current shade, go just two shades lighter than your natural base color, and you'll be collecting compliments about how Y&H you look. That's because "hair that's too dark emphasizes the lines on your face by throwing darkness into them," says Brad. "Severe dark color will age you." You can lighten up the strands that frame your face even more than two shades with highlights, the makeup you never take off. You'll create a halo of warmth — brightening up your face, illuminating your skin tone, and giving you an all-over glow.

No wonder so many actresses, singers, politicians, and news anchors have lightened up over the years, often going all the way to blond. Just look at Jane Fonda, Diane Keaton, Bette Midler, Barbra Streisand, Madonna, Hillary Clinton, Barbara Walters, and Katie Couric. Their blondness makes them look more luminous and glamorous, giving them a goddesslike glow in the light of the camera. Brad has lightened up the locks of Natasha Richardson, Brooke Shields, and Christy Turlington, as well as women who don't face the paparazzi daily but know that taking control of their color is powerful ammo in the war against aging.

Hair color is the first thing someone notices about you. So think about what your hair color is saying about you right now. If you're already coloring your hair, you've joined the majority of American women (54 percent of us) who realize that hair color can subtract ten years from our looks. At $10 a box, hair color is the original cheap ticket to looking younger. Here's to having fabulous hair color!

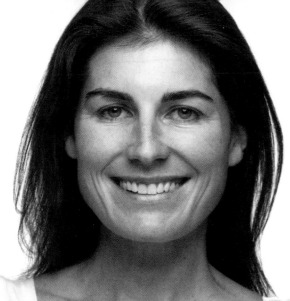

TOO OLD: Suzy before color

IT'S NOT ABOUT LOOKING NATURAL; IT'S ABOUT LOOKING FABULOUS

It's hard to believe that back in the fifties, hair color was such a big secret that "only her hairdresser knew for sure." Today the pressure is off. Your hair color doesn't have to be real. In fact, you don't win any points for being natural. Hair color is fashion, and the look of the moment is shiny, expensive color. It's a status symbol, not unlike a designer bag. Y&H color is more dramatic than natural color. "It's not about looking natural. Natural is boring," opines Brad. "It's all about being bright, bold, and expensive-looking." Although it doesn't actually have to be expensive, because at-home hair color is better than ever.

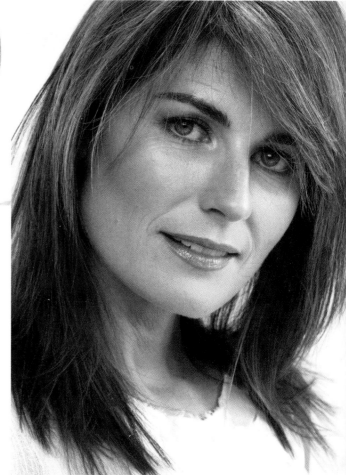

JUST RIGHT: Suzy lightened up by Brad

SHADES TO DYE FOR

Y&H color is not a simple, solid block of color, but multitonal, a well-designed range of color within the perfect shade. It's also about adding highlights around your face and going darker toward the back. Color, like everything else in life, is best done in moderation, so it's best to take baby steps when you're first starting color. You can always ratchet it up later. The reason some colorists suggest bringing in pictures from when you were two years old is that you can't go wrong if you look at your original color and go two shades up or down from there. Dark brunettes will look beautiful with lighter highlights. Blondes should not go darker than when they were a kid. Starting with your hair color as a toddler is a safe way to ensure that your new hair color will complement your skin tone and eye color. If you were to go five or more shades lighter, you might look washed-out without makeup, because your skin tone and your hair color may no longer be a match. Another reason you don't want to do an extreme color change is that it can damage your hair, causing breakage, which will not give you a healthy, glossy Y&H look. Crazy color changes are better left to teens in their experimental stage. At your stage, you want to look elegant, classy, and, well, sane. "You can have fun with color, but it's not like you're picking out lip gloss," says Brad. Within your chosen shade, you may want subtle hints of gold or flashes of red or copper, but stay away from hints of ashy blond, as it can come off looking drab.

HIGH, MEDIUM, AND LOW MAINTENANCE . . . HAIR COLOR

Only 15 percent of American women are salon-only when it comes to hair color. Twice as many (30 percent) do it themselves. And the number of women who get their hair colored at a salon *and* at home is on the rise. Ten percent of us are what Clairol calls "dualists." Whether you color your hair at a salon or at home, how often you need touching up depends on how far you've traveled from your roots. If you're going from very dark to very light or vice versa, rather than just two shades up or down, your roots will be more noticeable as they grow out. So tone it down a bit if you don't wish to become an every-three-week slave to hair color. Whatever you decide, you have options based on what your Visa card can handle.

HIGH: Top-of-the-line color czars in major cities can charge as much as $200 for a single-process color and $350 for highlights. To justify a scary $550 charge (not including tips), it's comforting to amortize the cost per day, because after all, hair color is the accessory you never take off. If you go for a root touch-up monthly and highlights seasonally (four times a year), you'll spend $3,800 a year on color. That's about $10 a day, roughly the cost of three lattes at Starbucks. You need to cut down on your coffee consumption anyway, don't you?

MEDIUM: Go to an expensive colorist twice a year, or go to a less expensive (but well-trained) colorist more frequently. Here's your script: "I love the work you do, but I can see you only once or twice a year. What are my options?" Let the colorist figure out how to accommodate you. Possible scenarios: A few highlights just around your face. Or a subtle set of tiny highlights all over that will blend in when your hair grows out (rather than changing the base color). Or color your base tone at home every month ($120 a year) and get highlights at a salon four times a year ($1,400), which will set you back $1,520 a year, or about $4 a day. (That's one latte at Starbucks.) Or ask your colorist if there is someone at the salon whom he or she has trained but who is less expensive. Or, if you live outside the area and you ask nicely, some benevolent hair color pros may even write down the formula they used so you can take it to a salon near you. Most professionals want you to look good, so they are willing to help if they can.

LOW: Go pro at least once, then follow up at home with the shade and brand recommended by your colorist that won't muck up the work just done. Professionals have studied the color wheel; they understand how hair tones interact, blend, and reflect off one another and what colors work best with what skin tones. So take full advantage of their skill and experience, then see if you can follow the plan in your own bathroom. At-home kits have the same tools and chemicals as those used at a salon — and they have never been better, with revised formulas, easier-to-understand instructions, and better-fitting gloves. Keep your color simple, and you'll save yourself a sinkful of cash.

A box of color once a month is $120 a year . . . a steal at less than a dollar a day . . . a mere 30 cents or so — far less than a cup of Starbucks coffee!

ARE YOU A SILVER FOX?

Choosing gray as a color (rather than going gray as a default option) can make a strong and powerful statement: you're old enough to carry an AARP card and don't give a damn who knows it! If you are in a position of power at, say, a Fortune 500 company, a law firm, a university, or Congress, and communicating your authority, experience, and gravitas serves your image better than looking youthful does, you may be tempted to become an elegant silver fox. Flaunting your gray in a "Youth R Us" culture takes guts — and commitment. If

If You Want to Go Gray

■ **Go virtually gray first.** Check out "The Newer Way to . . . Test-Drive Color" (opposite page). Put yourself in a gray head at clairol.com.

■ **Consult your colorist** and plan a time to let your roots grow out when you don't have a big event coming up. In three months, you will have two inches of gray roots. Adding highlights every few months will lighten your hair to decrease the contrast between the roots and your hair color.

■ **Cut your hair shorter.** Long, straggly hair is not the look you want. At least, chop off the ends.

■ **Shampoo with special products** to get rid of all yellow-toned strands (see Brilliant Buys). "Gray hair picks up yellow from hard water, the sun, and other products," says Brad Johns. "That's why you need a tinted shampoo once a month to cancel out the yellow." If you were blond as a child, you are likely to have white, not silver, hair. If you were brunette as a child, your hair will turn silver. Either way, yellow tones — the ultimate OL hair color no-no — must go.

■ **Condition your hair** with moisturizing and clarifying conditioners to make dry, brittle hair soft, smooth, and luxurious.

If You Don't Want to Go Gray

■ **When grays first debut,** it's easy to color them away at home with portable quick fixes. Two to try: Color Mark, a liquid temporary hair color that comes in a mascara-like wand in twelve shades. And Quick Tint, a twist-pen that comes in ten shades and washes out with one shampoo; and can also be used on a few stray brow hairs that are gray or white. (See Brilliant Buys.)

■ **Cover a few gray hairs yourself** at home with a semipermanent or demipermanent color in your base shade. This will darken the gray and blend it in. Clairol Natural Instincts is demipermanent and washes out after about twenty-eight shampoos.

■ **At a salon, you can ask for** strategically placed highlights to camouflage the gray.

■ **If you already have a single-process color** and gray roots are starting to show up before you can get to the salon, a genius product such as Clairol Nice 'N Easy Root Touch-Up will allow you to target just the roots with a tool that looks like a small paintbrush.

■ **Once you've gone more than 50 percent gray,** these kinds of easy fixes aren't going to look as good as coloring your base tone and touching up your roots every four to six weeks, which can be done at a salon or at home.

you dare to be a hair color rebel, know that going gray is not an easy pass to no-maintenance hair for the rest of your life. The best-looking manes of gray are those that shine like silver, sterling, platinum, pewter, or ice — and they probably get enhancing boosts from a colorist (as well as plenty of products to soften and shine). Looking glam with silver hair also requires an edgy haircut that's not past the shoulders, a killer body, and a sophisticated personal style, including compensatory chic clothes in the right shades and updated makeup that won't wash out your skin tone. Silver hair color requires high-maintenance grooming, because you are always trying to counteract the OGL (old gray lady) stereotype. If you let one thing go — for instance, if your hair is a mess, your outfit looks sloppy, or your makeup isn't done — you can look frumpy fast.

Is gray the new blond? My friend Lois Joy Johnson, beauty and fashion director of *More* magazine, thinks yes: "I think we're going to see a whole new generation of women who are going to make gray chic. It's not about letting yourself go. Going gray is a strategy. It's a power thing. It's not about being a granny." Lois points out how terrific Helen Mirren looked receiving her Oscar in 2007. "This woman does not seem like she had a stylist telling her what to do!" Lois says. Gray says you're in charge. But the first thing you need to take charge of is your transition to gray. You'll want to pull it off with panache. (See opposite page.)

The Newer Way to . . .

Test-Drive Color

In the old days, if you were feeling invisible and wanted to test the hair color waters before plunging in, you would trot off to a wig shop, play around with colors and styles, and assess the reaction from your mother, girlfriends, husband, and coworkers. Now you can buy inexpensive colored pieces from Hair Do (see chapter 2). But the newer way to explore

Better Blond!

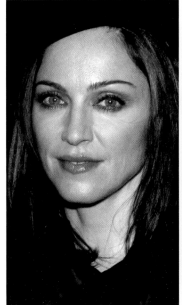
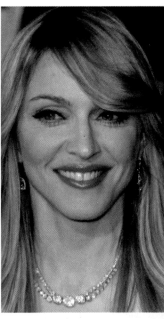

Madonna

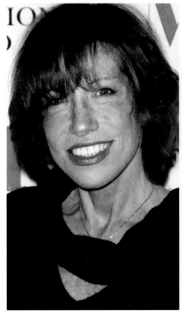
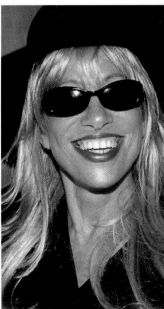

Carly Simon

Talking the Talk: Color

Describing color in words can be difficult. It's like telling a house painter, "I want my walls to be white." The paint store must have more than one hundred shades of white. That's why Brad Johns suggests using the universal language of food to describe color.

If you ask for:	You'll get hair the color of:
BLONDES	
Buttery	**Butter**
Golden	**Yellow mustard**
Butterscotch	**Butterscotch candy**
REDHEADS	
Strawberry blond	**Apricot jelly**
Medium red	**Paprika**
Auburn	**Cinnamon**
BRUNETTES	
Caramel	**A Kraft caramel**
Toffee	**The inside of a Heath bar**
Chocolate	**A Hershey's chocolate Kiss**
Coffee	**Coffee without cream**
Espresso	**Darker than coffee**
Black	**Licorice**

the subtleties of color and technique doesn't involve leaving your home. On the Web site clairol.com, you can upload your photo and try out the spectrum of shades on your own head. A brilliant way to see if you really want to go gray. (Warning: It's addictive!) If you want an expert opinion on one of your new looks, you can call one of Clairol's hair pros for a free phone consultation.

FINDING A COLORIST "TO MARRY"

To me, a woman's hair color is only as good as her colorist. The arrangement with my first colorist (my mother) couldn't have been more convenient, and the price was certainly right. But no offense, Mom, I would never let you near my head with rubber gloves today. When it comes to hair color, too many women opt for convenience over their best color possible, which is a unique formula based on equal parts shade, technique, and artistry. I know this sounds lofty, but the best colorists are truly artists, and the best cutters are masters of precision. That's why your hair colorist and haircutter should be a team, not the same person. A colorist who cuts your hair is not the best cutter, and a cutter who colors your hair is not the best colorist.

Women from the same town tend to look the same because they all go to the same colorist. This is another reason not to choose a colorist whose best attribute is location, location, location. Branch out; drive downtown. Some high-maintenance women even hop a plane and enjoy a beauty/shopping/theater weekend planned around their color appointments.

Search for your color soul mate the same way you would for any local beauty pro. When you see a woman on the street whose color you love, stop her and say, "I love your color. Where do you have it done?" Hopefully, she will be flattered and happy to share. You can also read beauty magazines, and make sure to check out "Getting Gorgeous City by City" in chapter 19 to find a great colorist in a city near you. If you get three confirmations that a colorist is the best around, start what Brad Johns calls "the dating process."

■ **The Coffee Date.** This is the first date, otherwise known as a consultation. Some colorists may charge $25 or so for a ten-minute consult. Before you let this person touch your hair, you need to know that you share the same values, at least in hair color. If he or she has crazy color, run. Even if a widely acknowledged "artist" thinks her hair looks pretty in pink, you're not on the same page color-wise. Speaking of pages, tear some out of magazines, showing color you love. Come armed with your own baby pictures, because going back to your roots is a very good place to start. The colorist should show you a portfolio of his or her work or photos of color he or she likes, but not shades from a color chart, because that's not how color looks on a person. If you have a good feeling after the coffee date, make dinner plans.

■ **The Dinner Date.** You're in the swivel chair. You love the color. But don't rush it. Live with the color for a few days before you decide to see the colorist again. Or, if you don't like the color, ask for a free redo. If you don't like the redo, keep dating.

■ **The Weekend Getaway.** After this second rendezvous, you'll know whether the colorist is The One to settle down with. If you love your color just as much this time, you're ready to commit. If not, continue the search.

■ **The Marriage.** It's your third time together, so you should feel very comfortable with this person by now. From this day forward, you may be seeing each other a lot, depending on your roots and your bank account. If you can't afford to see

Other Color To-Dos

✔**Protect Your Investment**

Now that you're invested in color, you want it to last. This means using shampoos and conditioners created especially for color-treated hair (see Brilliant Buys). Since color can be drying, these products are formulated to give color-treated hair extra moisture and not to overly strip the hair with detergent. I know this sounds like marketing spin, but these products are actually milder and more buffered than standard shampoos and conditioners. And don't use them every day; go a few days between washings. It's best if you can get away with washing your hair just twice a week.

✔**Be Proactive**

Summer sun and chlorine can do a number on your hair color. To maintain your color and luster, get fanatic about spritzing on a spray with UV protection designed especially for hair (see Brilliant Buys) and wear a cute straw hat when you're at the beach or pool, gardening, or outside for any stretch of time. If you're a swimmer, wet your hair with water from a sink, shower, or hose before you dip into the pool. Dry hair absorbs the liquid it first comes into contact with, and you don't want it to grab chlorine.

Buy a bathing cap, especially if you're a blonde. You didn't go through all that effort for your hair to turn green. Don't buy an OL cap with flower appliqués; Speedo has many sleek versions like the ones worn by Olympic athletes. When you're out of the pool, rinse your hair immediately with water, the more bubbly the better.

✔**Be Seasonal**

Just as you adapt your wardrobe to the time of year, adjust your hair color to reflect the light in winter, spring, summer, and fall. Even if you live where it's warm all year, a slight change with the seasons will prevent you from getting stuck in a rut and keep people guessing. In the summer, you should be at your lightest and brightest, so add more highlights. In the winter, you should be darker and richer, to match the heavier fabrics you're wearing, so use highlights more sparingly or make sure they, too, are in richer, warmer tones.

Talking the Talk: Process

You'll have a better chance of getting what you want from your colorist (or a box) if you speak the language.

Base color: Your overall hair color, natural or not.

Single process: The application of a permanent dye to change your base color up to six shades.

Double process: The rarely done procedure for changing your base color more than six shades, usually from dark to light. In the first process, the hair is stripped of its natural color. In the second, new color is deposited with a permanent dye. The two-step process is tricky and falls under the "do not try this at home" category.

Semipermanent color: A dye containing neither ammonia nor peroxide that does not lighten your hair color but can take a limited amount of gray two shades darker. Used primarily to enhance your natural color, it merely coats the hair with a new shade that washes out after about ten shampoos.

Permanent color: A dye used when you're more than 50 percent gray to change your hair color. It uses ammonia and peroxide to interact with the hair's inner structure and has the potential to damage hair if poorly applied, but it is also the only way to cover gray completely or to take hair more than two shades lighter (or darker). The color lasts until your hair grows out (or the colored strands are cut). Requires root touch-ups every four to six weeks.

Highlights: The Y&H essential that gives you that "I just came back from the beach" glow. Permanent lightener is applied to individual strands to create contrast with your base color, adding multiple dimensions of lightness.

Glaze: A semipermanent color placed on the hair for a short time to change tonality and add shine. To maintain the effect, the glaze needs to be reapplied every few weeks.

JUST RIGHT: Face-framing highlights from Brad give Michelle her all-over glow.

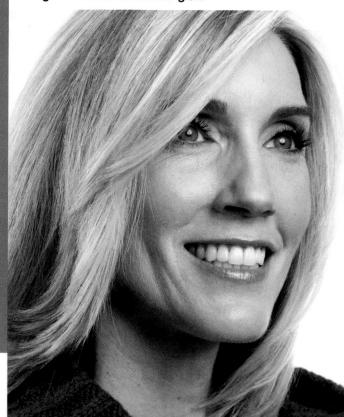

each other with the regularity your roots require, have a heart-to-heart about finances (see medium maintenance on page 25). And be prepared to be stopped on the street by women who want to know who does *your* color!

FOILED AGAIN

Even with all your dedication, you could end up with a hair color disaster. Rest assured, it happens to the best of us, even those who have a longtime colorist they know and love. Stay calm; don't scream. Even a permanent color mistake can be corrected. Go back to whoever did it and explain why you're unhappy. The colorist should redo it for free. (Some salons will do free redos up to seventy-two hours afterward, others up to two weeks.) If it's not right after the first redo, ask the salon for your money back or if you can be compensated with other salon services (manicures, massages, facials, etc.). If your longtime colorist doesn't fix it on the first try, take this as a sign that it's not a good match and the marriage is over. Don't you just love dating?

B R I L L I A N T   B U Y S

SHAMPOOS AND CONDITIONERS FOR COLOR-TREATED HAIR
Pantene Pro-V Expressions Color-Enhancing Shampoo, $5.99; and Conditioner, $5.99; drugstores and mass retailers

John Frieda Sheer Blonde Highlight Activating Shampoo, $6.49; and Conditioner, $6.49; drugstores and mass retailers

John Frieda Brilliant Brunette Shine Release Shampoo, $6.49; and Conditioner, $6.49; drugstores and mass retailers

L'Oréal Paris VIVE Pro Color Vive Shampoo; $4.99, and Conditioner, $4.99; drugstores and mass retailers

Clairol Nice 'n Easy ColorSeal Conditioning Gloss, $5; drugstores and mass retailers

SHAMPOOS AND CONDITIONERS FOR GRAY
Clairol Shimmer Lights Shampoo and Conditioner, $10.50; drugstores and mass retailers

L'Oréal Professionnel Colorist Collection White Violet Color Shampoo, $15; for salons, see lorealprofessionnel.com

Phyto Phytargent Whitening Shampoo, $24; for salons, call 800-55-PHYTO or phyto.com

AT-HOME COLOR
Clairol Natural Instincts, $8.99; drugstores and mass retailers

Clairol Nice 'n Easy Gray Solution, $8.99; drugstores and mass retailers

Garnier Color Breaks, $7.29; drugstores and mass retailers

Garnier Nutrisse, $7.29; drugstores and mass retailers

L'Oréal Paris Superior Preference hair color, $9.49, drugstores and mass retailers

COLOR TOUCH-UPS
Clairol Nice 'n Easy Root Touch-Up, $6.99, drugstores and mass retailers

Quick Tint, $14.95; 888-873-6443 or quicktint.net

Color Mark, $19.95; colormarkpro.com

COLOR PROTECTORS
Speedo Latex Caps, $2.50; theswimstore.com

Kérastase Paris Voile Protecteur, $34, for salons, call 877-748-8357 or kerastase.com

Phyto Plage "L'Originale" Protective Beach Spray, $20, Sephora, 877-737-4672 or sephora.com

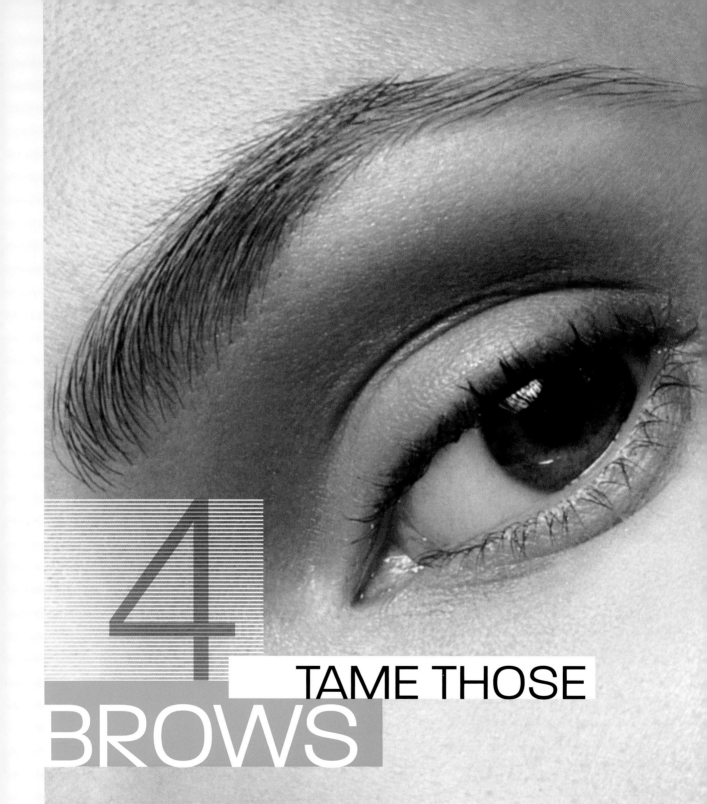

4

TAME THOSE
BROWS

NOTHING AGES YOU LIKE . . .
BUSHY, UNKEMPT EYEBROWS . . . SHAPELESS BROWS . . . TWEEZED-TOO-THIN BROWS . . . DRAWN-ON BROWS . . . GRAY BROW HAIRS

Let's give it up for great brows! They are the hardest-working — and most underappreciated — feature on your face. They really don't get the credit they deserve for their ability to transform your look. Because when they're good, they don't call attention to themselves. You notice the eyes, the lips, but rarely do you look at a woman and think, "Wow! She has the most gorgeous eyebrows." But what you *do* notice is how her whole face looks lifted. "It's the face-lift without the surgery," says Robert Sweet William, "the Brow Man" at Barneys New York, who has been artfully in charge of my brows for years. Of course, if the brows are bad, everyone will notice them. Bushy ones stick out like an angry line across your face. Unkempt ones make your face look dirty. Drawn-on brows make you look hard and severe. Too-thin brows do a disappearing act and leave your eyes without the proper framing.

A good brow has a classic, well-groomed shape that's timeless. It's true that different shapes and thicknesses come in and out of style, but those brows du jour should be saved for runway models and twentysomethings. As I'm writing this, it's all about the feral-looking full brow — a bushy look that seems to say, "I'm too young to own any tweezers." There's nothing Y&H about an unkempt brow on women our age. Even Brooke Shields (who's now in her forties) no longer has the full, bushy brows she made famous back in the eighties. Hers are now groomed into a very clean arch that will flatter her face for decades to come.

"As we get older, we need a more refined look," says Robert. "It's more sophisticated."

Makeup artists at fashion shows design the brows of the moment on models. Brow experts such as Robert maintain that real women shouldn't follow the trends: "People don't have the brows to go thick then thin, thick then thin. What I always tell my clients is, change your haircut, your color, your makeup, but the shape of your brows always stays the same." Amen.

Most of us probably couldn't grow bushy brows at this point anyway. As we age (sorry to repeat that phrase again), our brows naturally thin. Years of tweezing or waxing also take their toll and weaken the hair follicles. With these repeated assaults, the follicles scar, and the hairs grow back more slowly, if at all. Even in the best-case scenario, brow hairs take as long as six weeks to grow — a lot longer than the hair on your head. The point is, if you get too tweezer-happy, you may never see your brows again.

I've watched my mother deal with the daily maintenance of tweezer-induced browlessness. When she was nineteen and working at an insurance company in Chicago, a coworker did her the dubious favor of "fixing" her too-bushy brows. The problem is, she didn't just thin my mother's brows; she pulled out every single hair. To this day, my mother pencils in her brows with a Maybelline brow pencil before she leaves the house. Don't let this happen to you. Shape and groom your brows every time you do your makeup, but don't go crazy.

Tweezing Twicks

Since I'm medium maintenance when it comes to brows, I keep tweezers all over (cosmetic bag, drawers, bathroom shelves, glove compartment) and attend to stray hairs whenever I put on makeup. It's actually much easier than letting your brows go for several days, then trying to play catch-up. That's how you end up losing the shape and looking less-than-perfectly groomed. So stay on top of it, if you can. Here are some tricks to ease your pain.

■ **Invest in good tweezers.** Whether you choose slanted, flat, or pointed tips (I think slanted tips are best for grabbing hairs without poking the skin), your tweezers need to be sharp. Treat yourself to a better brand, such as Tweezerman.

■ **Tweeze after a shower.** The warmth of the water softens skin and relaxes pores, so hairs come out easier. Or press a warm washcloth directly on your brow before tweezing.

■ **Apply Anbesol.** This topical toothache anesthetic, applied to the brow about five minutes before tweezing, will numb the skin. When you're done, just wash it off.

■ **Give your brow a break.** Tweeze a few hairs from one brow, then switch to the other.

■ **Always pull in the direction of hair growth.** Hairs will be easier to extract.

GETTING A BROW-WOW SHAPE

What is your best brow shape and size? Although there is the classic brow — strong and well-defined, with a perfect arch — you also have to custom-shape your brows to fit your face. Some of us look better with a little more or less eyebrow depending on the size of our face, the shape of our eyes, and so on. No doubt you have encountered that convoluted pencil trick in magazines. This confusing method of determining your brow arch involves laying a pencil along the outside of your nose and seeing where it intersects with the inside of your eyebrow. Then you have to perform numerous calculations. Oh, please!

The Newer Way to . . .
Shape Your Brows

Buy an eyebrow stencil kit. I am a big fan of Senna Cosmetics Form-A-Brow Kit because it's goof-proof. If you can color in a picture in a kiddie coloring book, you can have wow brows. How? Choose the stencil (fine, natural, full, or extra full) that is closest to your real brow shape and line it up on your brow. Using the brow powder that best matches your brow hair (better to go too light than too dark), color inside the stencil. When you remove the stencil, the hairs that aren't colored — the ones that were outside the stencil — can be tweezed away. Now you've probably been told not to tweeze any hair from above the brow, but the experts agree that's a myth. If you have hairs that are ruining your perfect shape, let them go.

The other option, of course, is to put your brows in the hands of a professional. If you have the time and can find someone who really knows what he or she is doing, why not? Be forewarned: creating great eyebrows is an art, so don't entrust yours to just anybody. (Remember what happened to my mother!) Get a referral from a friend whose brows you love.

What's the best way to shape your brows and remove stray hairs? Reasonable people disagree, but the purists swear by tweezing, and I concur. Tweezers are precise and easy, and they fit in a makeup bag, so you can always have a pair at the ready. Many brow experts use a combination of tweezing and waxing to create the perfect shape. The downside of waxing is that it can be damaging (not to mention painful!) to the delicate, thin skin around the eyes. The upside is that it can remove a lot of hairs — including baby-fine strands tough to grab with tweezers — in a single swipe. The fact that it's so easy to take off a lot at once is why you should never wax your own brows. The third option is threading — an ancient Asian technique using a cotton thread that wraps around a row of hairs and pulls them out. Full disclosure: I have never been threaded. But Nora Ephron, in *I Feel Bad About My Neck,* describes it as "quick and painful (although not, I should point out, as painful as, say, labor)," with results that last about a month. Like waxing, this is not something you're going to do at home.

DAILY BROWSING

Now that your brows are in good shape, you're ready for part 2: Brows, The Sequel . . . filling them in with makeup. Even the best-shaped brows need to have those bare patches covered with a little bit of powder. I like to use stencils — fill them in with brow powder — and seal the deal with brow mascara (a product I can't live without).

If you don't have brow stencils, use a sharp eyebrow pencil to draw in "hairs" where there aren't any — but be sure to use short, feathery strokes that mimic the look of the real thing. Then take a stiff, slanted eyebrow brush and use it to

Other Brow To-Dos

✔**Banish Bulk**
If you have naturally heavy brows, just shaping may not be enough. The best way to eliminate excess fullness is to trim brow hairs. Use an eyebrow brush to sweep hairs upward. Trim any that extend up beyond where you want your brows to end with small brow scissors.

✔**Avoid Silly Shapes**
The two worst shapes are brows that are too rounded (clownlike — the top half of a circle) and those that are too paisley (where the inner corner is thick, then the brow thins out). Neither of these is flattering. The ideal brow has a similar, moderate thickness throughout, tapering just slightly at the outer corner. Keep the tail long — it's younger-looking.

✔**Add Color**
If you color your hair a shade that's far from your natural one, color your brows as well. Blondes should have brows just a shade darker than their hair, brunettes the same shade or a shade lighter, and redheads the same shade or a shade darker. In some states (New York, for example), it's illegal to have permanent dye applied to your brows, although every salon I've been to will do it if you ask. Should you decide to do it at home, err on the side of caution: keep the dye on for only a minute or two at most.

✔**Cope with Grays or Whites**
I know it's tempting to just tweeze these out, especially when there is only one or two. But it's a bad habit to start tweezing out hairs just because of their color. Better to use a brow pencil, brow powder, or hair dye instead.

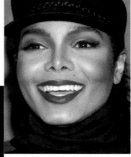

Brows too bushy

JUST RIGHT: Janet Jackson's defined brows lift her face.

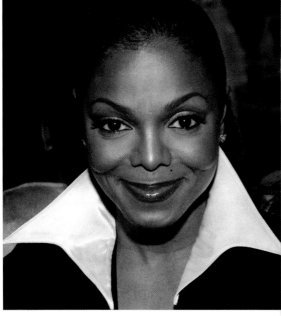

apply brow powder to give your brows more definition. The last step is to set brows with a sweep of clear brow gel or tinted brow mascara. Use it sparingly (and wipe off any excess with a cotton swab dipped in eye makeup remover) to avoid any dandruff-like flakes.

Brows too dark

JUST RIGHT: Sarah Jessica Parker's matching brow color makes all the difference.

small tweak can have a big impact on your Y&H factor.

HIGH: Leave these matters in the hands of professionals. Schedule standing appointments six months out with the best brow guru in town. Every three weeks, you'll spend just fifteen minutes in the chair, and you'll see what a difference a great brow makes. The going rate: $25 to $65 per visit.

MEDIUM: Seek professional help when you've lost your shape (every six weeks or so), and splurge for special occasions. Between visits, DIY.

LOW: DIY. Do your own. Armed with good tweezers and a magnifying mirror, a brow pencil, powder, and a stencil, you can do it!

HIGH, MEDIUM, AND LOW MAINTENANCE . . . GREAT BROWS

Beautiful brows can be yours, no matter what your level of dedication to the cause. Just don't ignore them. They are the only feature on your face that you can easily change, and even a

Brow Fixes: Extensions, Prosthetics, and Tattooing

Some women experience a loss of brow hairs due to injury, illness, or even waxing or tweezing mishaps. If you do not have enough hairs to create a lush brow with a pencil and powder, you may want to investigate temporary brow enhancements, such as extensions or prosthetics. LuxLash in Boston offers brow extensions — individual synthetic brow hairs that are applied to your own in the same way that lash extensions are. The ninety-minute process starts at $100, and the results can last for up to four weeks. If your brows are too sparse, a brow prosthetic is a synthetic brow applied to your face with an adhesive. These start at $250, are reusable, and can last for years. (See "Your Go-To List" in chapter 19.) If your brow loss is permanent, the best solution might be cosmetic tattooing, which can cost $550 or more. Though long lasting, the color will fade to purple and will require maintenance touch-ups. To find a salon specializing in this, go to the Web site of the Society of Permanent Cosmetic Professionals (spcp.org). Big warning from Robert Sweet William of Barneys New York, who has seen his share of tattoos gone wrong: "Make sure you really want to do this, and do this only if you really need it." Because it's permanent, it's more critical than ever that you do the research to find a gifted tattoo artist. Aside from getting a good recommendation, his advice is, "Make sure you see people [the artist has] done who have been done well." Got it.

B R I L L I A N T   B U Y S

TWEEZERS
Tweezerman Slant Tweezer, $20; Tweezerman, 800-645-3340 or tweezerman.com

BROW PENCILS
Kevyn Aucoin Beauty The Precision Brow Pencil, $24; kevynaucoin.com
Lancôme Le Crayon Poudre, $23; Saks, 877-551-7257; lancome.com
Maybelline New York Expert Eyes Brow & Eye Liner, $5.79; drugstores and mass retailers
Senna Cosmetics Brow Shaper Pencil, $16; Senna Cosmetics, 800-537-3662 or sennacosmetics.com

BROW POWDER
Paula Dorf 2 + 1 for Brows, $24; pauladorf.com

BROW STENCILS
Senna Cosmetics Form-A-Brow Kit, $42; Senna Cosmetics, 800-537-3662 or sennacosmetics.com

BROW MASCARA
Senna Cosmetics Brow Fix, $18; Senna Cosmetics, 800-537-3662 or sennacosmetics.com

BROW KITS
Anastasia All About Brows Kit, $75; Sephora, 877-737-4672 or sephora.com
Chanel Sourcils Duo Professionnel, $35; Saks, 877-551-7257; saks.com

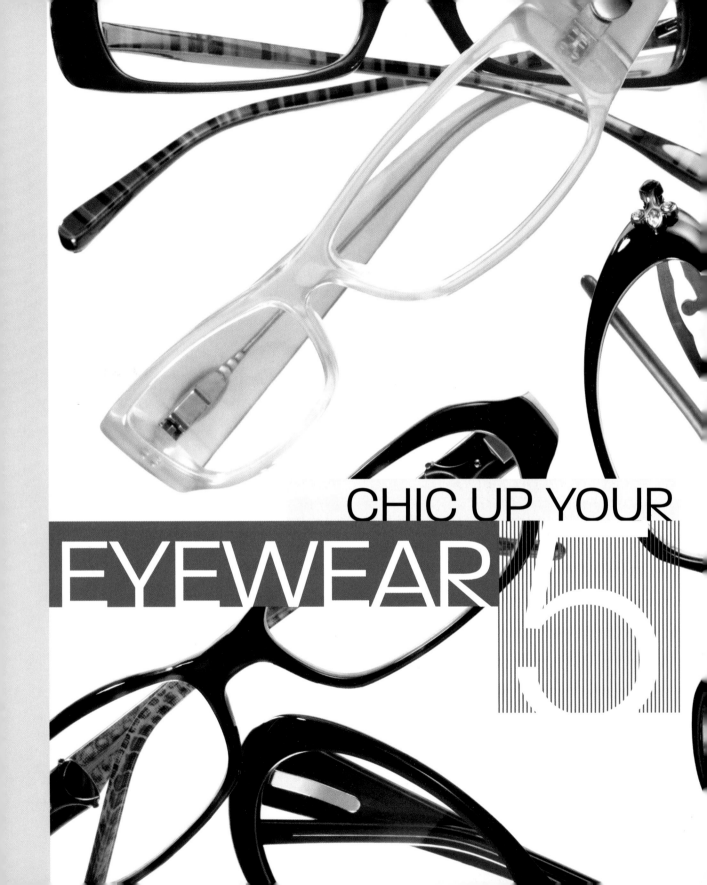

CHIC UP YOUR
EYEWEAR 5

NOTHING AGES YOU LIKE ...
DATED FRAMES ... BORING FRAMES ... FRAMES THAT DROOP DOWNWARD ... METAL RIMS ... RIMLESS GLASSES ... HALF-GLASSES ... AN EYEGLASS NECKLACE ... BIFOCALS ... COKE-BOTTLE LENSES ... SQUINTING

t's a cliché in Hollywood movies that when a woman transforms from a buttoned-up Ms. Priss to a bursting-with-passion temptress, she does two things: unpins her fussy, Marian-the-librarian bun and whips off her owlish Coke-bottle eyeglasses. This particular cliché has two morals: (1) If you don't have to wear glasses, don't. With either LASIK surgery or contact lenses, you can ensure that people have an unobstructed view of your beautiful eyes. (2) If you do need glasses (as most of us do), make sure they are sexy and cool, not anything that Marian the librarian would wear.

It's amazing how a few sculpted ounces of plastic or metal can make an instant impression about your style. Glasses can make you look edgy, intriguing, artsy, intellectual, or authoritative. Just think of Meryl Streep in *The Devil Wears Prada*. Off camera, actresses such as Liv Tyler and Nicole Kidman have whipped out sexy eyeglasses at awards shows to read the teleprompter and instant-messaged the world, "Not only am I gorgeous, but I'm smarter than you think."

Oprah once dedicated a show to how changing "just one thing" can make a huge difference in your look. For my segment on the show, I stood in Rockefeller Center in Manhattan and pulled aside women wearing outdated eyeglass frames. I took them into a cool eyewear boutique and gave them an update. Wow! What a difference just that one change made. Because of their prominence on the face, eyeglasses can have a powerful impact. After all, they're visible all day long. More important than any other fashion accessory, glasses stay with you until you're ready for bed. They can make or break your look, so be sure they say, "This woman has style!"

If you need convincing to update your eyewear (see the list below), think about the most important reason to get new glasses: your eye health. Doctors recommend that all those over forty get their eyes checked at least once a year (more often if you start to have vision problems). If you can't remember the last time you had your

Top Five Reasons to Change Your Eyewear

1. You may need a new prescription.
2. You have a new job or a promotion.
3. You broke your glasses. (The safety pin trick is not an option.)
4. You changed your hair color.
5. You need to use up extra money from your flexible spending account. (Read more about this later in the chapter.)

vision checked, chances are your prescription has changed. Sure, this probably means your eyes have gotten worse, but what a great excuse to hip up your look. Don't even *think* about putting new lenses in old frames. The universe is sending you a chance to be more fashion-forward; go with it!

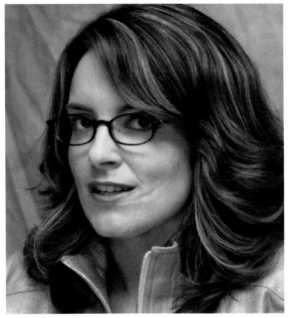

Tina Fey: a model of specs appeal

FRAMES ARE FASHION

So if you're still putting frames in the same category as kitchen appliances — functional, unsexy, and designed to be used for as long as they work — consider this: there isn't a big-name fashion house without its logo on a line of eyeglasses. We're talking Gucci, Prada, Dolce & Gabbana, Chanel, Michael Kors, Marc Jacobs, Vera Wang, Donna Karan, Badgley Mischka, Fendi, Giorgio Armani, Valentino, Moschino, Carolina Herrera, Coach, Kate Spade, and even Juicy Couture. And just like the fashion industry, eyeglass manufacturers launch new lines seasonally. Every spring and fall, they introduce new styles, shapes, colors, and technology. Wearing frames that are five years old is like wearing shoes that are five years old: they may serve their basic purpose, but are they going to make you look current? No.

Eyewear (like makeup and fragrance) is an accessible way to get in on the ground floor of a luxury label and own a piece of your favorite designer. When you look at the big picture of all things designer, frames are not outrageously priced. As you well know, the latest Prada bag can easily set you back $1,500 at Neiman Marcus, but the latest Prada eyewear can be yours for just $220 at LensCrafters. When you do the fashion math, designer eyewear is a steal. And although a Gucci gown might be cut too sexy, Gucci glasses will fit.

YOUR WARDROBE OF FRAMES

Designer names, seasonal collections, up-to-the-minute trends, and cutting-edge technology: frames are fashion. And just as you have the appropriate shoes, bags, and clothing to wear to work, on weekends, and to a black-tie benefit dinner, shouldn't you have appropriate glasses to wear to each of these as well?

The eyewear industry has been trying for years to convince us that we need a wardrobe of glasses. Yes, they're trying to increase sales, but I think they have a point. Obviously, having a wardrobe of glasses makes more sense if you need them all the time. If you need them solely for driving or for going to the movies, well, lucky you; you can get by with one pair of chic frames. But if you have them on your face all day, every day, you may want to vary your look from time to time. I know, glasses are really expensive. The last time I bought a pair, I walked out with a $1,200 bill. (I'll tell what I've learned later in this chapter.) But if you can afford to stock your eyeglass wardrobe, do it!

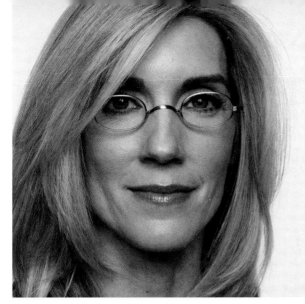

TOO OLD: granny glasses

What You Need in Your Wardrobe

There are three main scenarios for which you need a great pair of glasses: at work, on the weekend, and for dressy occasions.

■ **For the office,** get a shape and color that looks stylishly professional. You want to look polished, not kooky.

■ **On the weekend,** you can unleash the real you with wilder frames in a striking color such as bright white, red, or pink or a leopard, zebra, or giraffe print.

■ **For formal occasions,** wow them with a pair of glamour glasses. Look for temples and logos detailed in jewels, crystals, or pearls from designers such as Valentino, Chanel, Dior, and Judith Leiber, who makes frames to match her legendary evening bags (that is, embedded with cabochon stones, authentic mother-of-pearl, or Austrian crystals).

Now that you know what you want in your wardrobe of glasses, here's what's OL. Don't put anything on your face that you'd be likely to see on a high school math whiz or a nun. These include rimless glasses (too grandma); thin, gold, metal frames (too boring); and round, Harry Potter–type frames (too collegiate). Also steer clear of adornments such as ornamen-

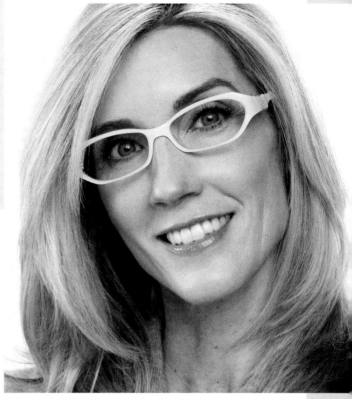

JUST RIGHT: a cool pair that's Y&H

tal leaf or flower patterns (too nerdy). If Betty Suarez on TV's *Ugly Betty* would wear them, they're not for you.

PUTTING YOUR OLD GLASSES TO GOOD USE

I used to have an entire drawer in my closet dedicated to old eyewear, taking up valuable real estate. Why? Maybe it was an emotional attachment; maybe it was the money I had spent on them. But as my mother would say, they owed me nothing. My eyes outgrew those prescriptions, and as for the frames, trust me, even if they did come back in style, new technology would render them old

If it's on your body, and headed south, it needs to make a U-turn.

and dated. Rather than just tossing your glasses, however, be good to yourself and someone else by donating them. Lions Clubs worldwide collect more than five million pairs of used glasses a year, repair them, and distribute them to people who need them. (Go to lionsclubs.org to find a drop-off location near you.) Or visit your local LensCrafters, where employees will accept any pair of glasses and donate them to people in developing countries. (See lenscrafters.com for details.) Done!

FINDING YOUR PERFECT FRAMES

In this book, certain principles cut across all categories. **Principle 1:** Defy gravity. To look younger, everything that can be hoisted upward, must be — breasts, butt, neck, brows, eyes. If it's on your body, and headed south, it needs to make a U-turn. Your eyeglass frames are no exception. That's why you'll look better in frames that are horizontal, with a slight upward tilt at the outer edges. Avoid any that slope down on the sides. Down-turned frames will make your face look droopy, saggy, and sad. Upturned frames, like a sexy cat eye, will draw the eye upward and accentuate your cheekbones. Love that!

Principle 2: Bring warmth, color, and softness to your face. When choosing frames, opt for high-quality European plastic (zyl) in a tortoiseshell, color, or translucent over cold, icy metal.

Beyond these two principles, eyewear professionals over the years have suggested a multitude of factors to consider when buying frames, including face shape, face size, eye color, hair color, skin tone, makeup, predominant wardrobe color, personal style statement, fit, and budget. It's enough to make you dizzy before trying on one pair.

Put all these things out of your mind, set aside a few hours, and go to a store with a selection of top-tier designer frames. Find somebody who has some style to help you, then try and try and try. When you put on the right pair, you will just know it; it's like finding the right house. The perfect frame will elevate you to the next style level and bring out your best features. If you can't choose between two frames and you're high maintenance, buy both. If you're not high maintenance, decide which frames will go the distance with your wardrobe. You don't want to invest in, for instance, a red frame if your wardrobe consists of yummy shades of orange (or vice versa).

Why not go to the best in the biz when it comes to eyewear? **Welcome to your consultation with eyewear king Robert Marc.**

In New York City, the name Robert Marc is synonymous with the latest and greatest in eyewear. You'll find his eponymous line of frames at his own chic boutiques in Manhattan's hottest shopping spots. He also has a place in Boston. But wherever you live, you'll find Robert Marc frames at the hippest eyewear boutiques worldwide.

Robert says his first hard-and-fast rule is that the frame be in proportion to your face and features. So if the current craze is for enormous frames but your face is small, find oversized frames that are in balance with your face. How will you know this? For one thing, see where the frames hit your eyebrow. "The top of a frame should be at the bottom of the brow, but not over it," Robert says. "We do not want to see the brow in the lens."

As for the practice of choosing frames to fit the shape of the face, Robert says, "When it comes to face shape, most of the advice is from books written in the 1950s." Face shape is a factor, but don't follow it off a cliff, because some of the newer frames might look great on you even if they are not the obvious shape for your face. That said, the most flattering frames just may be those that counterbalance the shape of your face. So if your face is round, try rectangular frames with sharp or right angles. If your face is more square, choose frames with softer curves.

If you've achieved the proper balance in the frames, Robert says the second most important factor is choosing the right color. How the frames blend with your hair color is more important than how they match your eye color or the prevailing color in your wardrobe. Tortoiseshell frames are almost universally flattering because they include so many tonalities found in hair color and come in an endless variety of shades and undertones. "Except for black, which is chic and smart on virtually everyone, I like warmer colors on women," Robert says. He favors reds, oranges, browns, and burgundies over cool colors such as blues, grays, and antique silver, which can be aging.

Even within the warmer tones, there is a carnival of color out there, and selecting the right one can be daunting. Apply Robert's rules of hair color.

• **If you have blond hair:** Whites and translucents tend to look good on blondes. Or go with a medium-tone brown or tortoiseshell that has a predominantly olive, yellow, or rose undertone. Conventional wisdom says that black is too harsh for blondes, but I have a pair of shiny, black Chanels, and they're the chicest pair I've ever owned.

• **If you have red hair:** Opt for a warm brown or tortoiseshell. Avoid anything too yellow in favor of rich henna tones.

• **If you have brown hair:** A deep brown, burgundy, or golden-hued tortoiseshell will look smashing.

• **If you have black hair:** Select a black or a non-yellow tortoiseshell. If your hair is blue-black, go with a dark brown that has no yellow or red.

• **If you have gray hair:** Choose red or burgundy to add color. This is the one hair color that tends to clash with tortoiseshell, as the pattern is often too yellow to be flattering.

Don't try to match frames to your eye color. Instead, Robert says it's important to get an antireflective coating on the lenses so that people can see through them to your eyes. Also, you'll look better wearing eye makeup. Lipstick, too, is important. "You're adding color and volume to the top of your face when you're wearing glasses," Robert says. "To balance the top of the face with the bottom, you need a great pair of lips."

HIGH, MEDIUM, AND LOW MAINTENANCE . . . SHOPPING FOR EYEWEAR

HIGH: Updating your eyewear every season is de rigueur. It's no different than buying new shoes and bags. You need a pair of glasses for the office, for the weekend, and for black-tie events. And then there are sunglasses, sports glasses, driving glasses, lazy-Sunday-afternoon glasses . . . Go to the chicest boutique in town and do one-stop shopping.

MEDIUM: Update only one category a year in your wardrobe of frames for work, play, and dressy occasions. Go to the chicest boutique in town to research the frames you want, then shop smart online. Bring the frames to your optician and have the lenses put in.

LOW: Buy one pair of super-chic glasses that serve all your needs. To save on the frames, buy hip reading glasses at a department store or specialty shop, bring them to the optician, and have your prescription popped in. To save on sunglasses, consider transitional lenses.

**Splurge on a wardrobe of eyewear.
For weekends:** fun shapes and colors

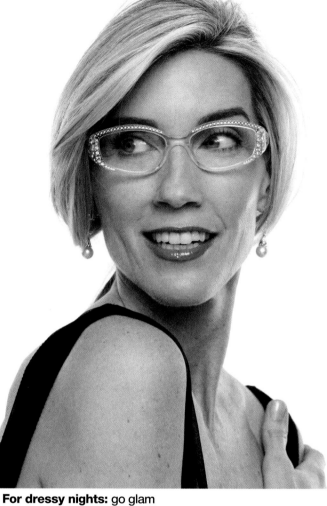

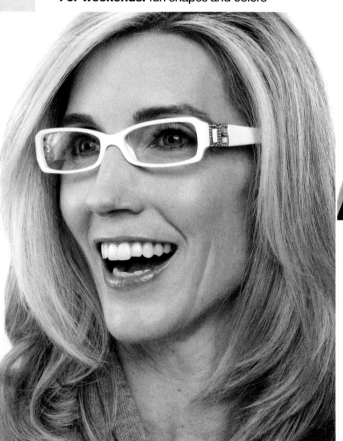

For dressy nights: go glam

THE LATEST IN LENSES

Frames are not the only part of your eyewear that may need a makeover. If your lenses are thick, have a clear line of demarcation between the top and bottom (that is, bifocals), or make your eyes look magnified, you are going to look OL. Fortunately, technology is on your side.

Extremely thick lenses are extremely passé,

so if your vision is really bad, ask for high-index lenses. These are made of a thinner and lighter plastic than traditional lenses, so even if you need a significant correction, you don't need to be sporting a wide wedge of lens. These babies don't come cheap. You'll probably end up paying about $215 for the lenses (roughly $90 more than the standard thick lenses), but they're worth it.

As we get older, usually starting around age forty, the lenses in our eyes get stiffer and less flexible, a condition known as presbyopia. This makes it harder for them to focus on things close up and makes it necessary for us to buy reading glasses, which magnify type read at close range.

What you want to avoid is traditional bifocals. The word alone conjures up images of blue-haired ladies sitting around a bingo table. But also, the visible line that separates the upper and lower parts of the lens deters people from looking at you, kid, and is a red flag of old age. Bifocals also tend to make the eyes look weirdly enormous, as if they were being seen through a magnifying glass. Progressive lenses, sometimes called "invisible bifocals," solve these problems. Instead of starkly separating the top portion of the lenses (dedicated to seeing distances) from the bottom portion (designed for reading), progressive lenses transition between the two invisibly. In fact, you can get trifocals, in which the two are separated by a middle area for seeing intermediate distances. The drawback is that these lenses can require an adjustment period. Also, some trendy narrow frames may not offer enough room to accommodate all three portions. Progressive lenses cost anywhere from $180 to $325 (about $80 more than traditional bifocals), but the cost of saving your dignity? Priceless.

SHOPPING SMART FOR EYEWEAR

By now, you no doubt have signed on to the idea of needing more than one pair of glasses, but before you refinance your mortgage to make it possible, check your insurance plan. Some acknowledge the fact that prescriptions change every year, particularly after age forty, and cover at least a portion of the cost of new glasses annually.

The other avenue to investigate is your flexible spending account (FSA). Some insurance plans allow people to set aside pretax dollars for health care costs, including prescription eyeglasses. In some cases, the money must be used within a year (although some plans extend the time frame to fourteen months), or it is forfeited. Buying glasses is a great way to use any money left over in your FSA. And that's the reason for the rush on frames in February.

Still another way to save money is to buy your frames and lenses separately when it makes sense. Many retailers would have you believe that the two must be bought together. Not true. So shop around for the best price on frames, but don't skimp on quality lenses. Manufacturers often sell frames to vendors without a suggested retail price, and the markup can vary dramatically from store to store. Much of the designer eyewear is licensed to one of the two Italian manufacturers of eyeglass frames — Luxottica or Safilo — and between them, they own LensCrafters, Pearle Vision, Sunglass Hut, and Solstice Sunglass Stores. That's why it's easier than ever to find the big designer names — Armani, Valentino, Gucci, Dior, Donna Karan, Versace — online or at a mall near you. You can also get great deals on top-of-the-line designer frames at discount retailers such as Costco. Just buy the frames there, bring them to your optician, and have the lenses put in.

You can find deals online if you search, but don't buy frames without trying them on first. It's impossible to tell how the shape and color will look on you based solely on a picture. If you want to shop online, do your in-person research, then see if you can find the same model on the Internet.

(PLEASE DON'T . . .)

Hang your eyeglasses from a necklace. No matter how bejeweled the necklace, it screams OL. (The Y&H aren't always forgetting where they put their glasses!) I admit that whenever I'm about to leave for the movies, I always ask, "Where did I put my glasses?" But I don't have to let the whole world know that. The better solution is to have a wardrobe of glasses stashed in various places: the glove compartment of your car, your desk drawer, your bedside table . . .

GOING WITHOUT: GLASSLESS OPTIONS

Yes, eyeglasses can make you look smart, sexy, and chic, but the quickest way to look Y&H is to wear no glasses at all. The most permanent solution is to get LASIK surgery, in which a laser is used to correct near- and farsightedness. This is a great option, but it's not for everyone, for a variety of reasons, including eye shape, astigmatism, and other eye problems. The only way to know for sure if it will work for you is to ask your eye doctor.

The other way to bid your specs adieu is to wear contact lenses, which offer an added bonus: you can get them tinted to add "va va va voom" to your eye color. Colored contact lenses are more wearable than ever, with colors that look more natural than they used to. Both Acuvue 2Colours and FreshLook ColorBlends get high marks. You can buy a box of six lenses for about $50. One pair can last from two to four weeks. Colored lenses can give you more eye drama. I sometimes pop Acuvue's green enhancers in before a special event, and what a difference!

You do, however, have to be careful not to look otherworldly. Have you ever looked into somebody's eyes and seen color so unnatural that she looks like a creature from another planet? It shouldn't be obvious that you're wearing colored contact lenses. It's worse when

SEXY SHADES

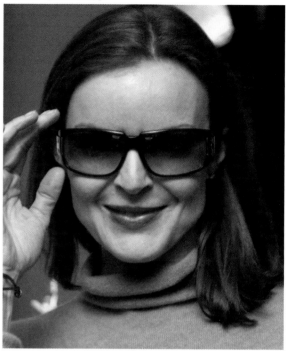

Marcia Cross

the color is not your natural one — meaning yesterday you showed up for work with blue eyes, and today they're brown. If the colored lenses don't match your own eye color in a natural way, check out enhancers. Enhancers are lenses with transparent pigment that amplify your own color. And you don't have to have bad eyesight to wear them. You can buy noncorrective ones if you simply want stunning eye color.

If you are super high maintenance and find such off-the-rack color choices too predictable, you can explore the possibility of custom color lenses. Dr. Mitch Cassel, who runs the Studio Optix shop in Rockefeller Center in Manhattan, creates one-of-a-kind contact lenses for actors and actresses to wear in movies. For a mere $1,250 he'll create a pair just for you.

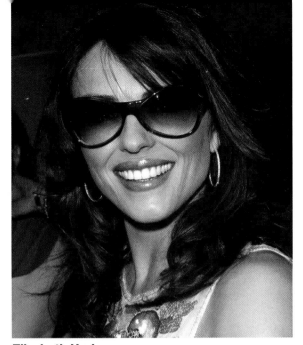

Elizabeth Hurley

HIP READERS:
ONE MORE WAY TO ACCESSORIZE

Many women freak out the first time they have trouble reading the back of a bottle of Advil. After all, losing the ability to see close up is a sure sign you're not a kid anymore. Slipping on a cool pair of readers is better than digging out a magnifying glass when you need to read tiny mouse type. Standard, over-the-counter readers come in various strengths (1–3) known as diopters. I started off needing a 1 and am now up to a 2.5. When you can no longer see clearly with a 3, it's time to see your eye doctor for a stronger prescription. Please don't settle for the crummy-looking generic kind you find at the drugstore checkout counter. Forget about those half-glasses, the Benjamin Franklin–type specs that sit on the edge of your nose or those connected by a raised nosepiece over the frames. Instead, buy full-frame readers that are so fun you'll never want to take them off. Corinne McCormack's fashion-forward readers are so trendy that they're sold in the accessories department at Bloomingdale's. "Women think that they can play games and squint and hold the paper further and further away," says Corinne,

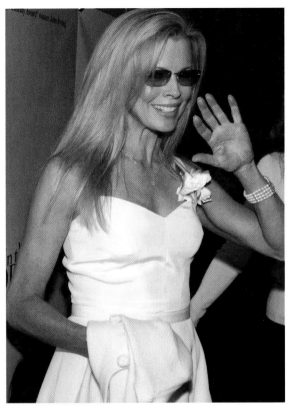

Kim Basinger

"but it's not good for your eyes or your face." And why wouldn't you want to wear glasses from Corinne's line, which are so witty and stylish (I love the 1950s-looking rhinestone detail) that women who don't need help with their vision are buying them anyway — and replacing the corrected lenses with clear ones for a sophisticated, fashionable business look. Katie Couric wears them on TV, and Judy Davis wore the "Hollywood" frame in the film *The Break-Up*. Since they cost only $48, you may want to buy a pair and have your eyewear professional pop in your regular prescription lenses. And since they're much less expensive than other glasses (because they come in standard, as opposed to prescribed, powers), you can afford to have multiple pairs stashed all over the house. But if you're anything like me, you'll still always be asking, "Where did I put my glasses?"

SUNGLASSES: INSTANT GLAMOUR

An easy way to pump up your sexiness quotient is to slip on a pair of large shades whenever you step out of the house — whether it's sunny or not. It's incredible how much glam you get from just a thin layer of plastic and a couple of pieces of hardware. You'll look mysterious and chic, plus it's a great way to shave time off your beauty regimen when you don't have a few extra minutes to put on eye makeup. Just remember not to take the sunglasses off when you meet someone you know (no matter how rude it may seem). Of course, there are important health reasons to slip on a pair of sexy shades. Sunglasses are sunblock for your eyes, shielding them from UV rays and warding off health issues such as macular degeneration and cataracts. With shades, you'll squint less, helping you keep crow's-feet and forehead wrinkles at bay, and you'll protect the delicate skin on

the sides of your eyes, just as long as you make sure the shades cover that area as well. It's key that sunglass lenses offer 100 percent UV protection (see "Is It Worth It?"). Don't assume that just because lenses are dark, they will block out dangerous rays.

With sunglasses, you're going for a different look, and therefore a different fit, than with your prescription glasses. Because you want them to protect the entire eye area rather than frame it, sunglasses can cover your eyebrows. Frames that might look too big with optical lenses can look hip with shades.

What's Hot Now

What's happening in eyewear, and particularly in sunglasses, reflects what's happening in fashion in color and style. When white is big in fashion, white shades are hot. You can never go wrong by checking out the shades of hot designers such as Chanel, Gucci, Dior, Fendi, and Dolce & Gabbana. They always get it right.

Always in fashion are wraparound shades. They're glamorous, and they cover the vulnerable skin around your eyes. They also offer a peripheral barrier from dust and wind.

Black frames and tortoiseshell frames look flattering with most people's coloring and go with everything. They should be a staple of your wardrobe, like a white shirt or a pair of jeans.

As for tinted lenses, the darker the better. Gray, green, and brown lenses are all excellent all-purpose tints, but stay away from yellow or pink lenses. For one thing, they can actually make the sun look brighter. For another, who wants to look like a drug addict? Worst of all, they can make you look like you're trying too hard, which, as you know by now, is so OL.

$ Is It Worth It?

Designer Sunglasses. Top designer sunglasses can run upwards of $300. You can buy a similar-looking pair from a sidewalk or flea market vendor or at a mall kiosk for $10. So should you spend the big bucks? Yes!

Go for quality over price, as the cheap ones are unlikely to protect your eyes from UV rays. Yes, sunglasses look great, but they also serve a very important purpose: protecting your corneas from the damaging effects of the sun. The lenses in sunglasses bought at optical shops or department stores likely have been treated to filter out UV rays. Look for a sticker reading "UV400," signaling that the lenses meet the requirement of blocking 99 percent of UV rays. A pair of $10 shades may stop you from squinting, but they may not really be protecting your eyes. You're worth a good pair of sunglasses — just don't leave them at the restaurant!

B R I L L I A N T   B U Y S

ON OPENER (PAGE 38) FROM TOP, CLOCKWISE

EYEWEAR
Corinne McCormack Emily Cherry readers, $48; Bloomingdale's, Lord & Taylor or corinnemccormack.com
Gucci Truffle translucent eyeglasses, GG2922, $250; for retail locations, Safilo, 800-772-2157
Badgley Mischka Eye Couture by Sama, "Victoria" frame, about $750; Robert Marc, 212-675-5200
Dolce & Gabbana Purple eyeglasses, DG3001, $270; LensCrafters, lenscrafters.com
Robert Marc Havana layered with Bamboo Snake, 177, $365; robertmarc.com or 212-675-5200

ON OUR MODEL

JUST-RIGHT FRAMES (PAGE 41):
Robert Marc Cream layered with Henna Snake, 177, $365; robertmarc.com or 212-675-5200

WEEKEND FRAMES (PAGE 44):
Dolce & Gabbana White with logo, DG3011, $300; LensCrafters or lenscrafters.com

DRESSY FRAMES (PAGE 44):
Ferragamo Clear with crystals, FE2625, $249; LensCrafters or lenscrafters.com

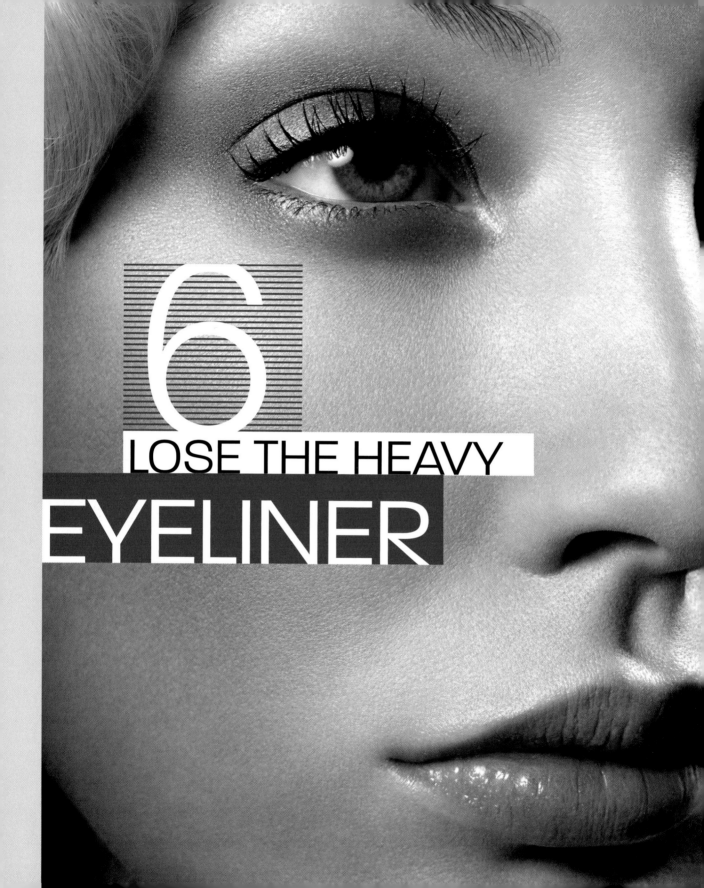

6

LOSE THE HEAVY
EYELINER

NOTHING AGES YOU LIKE...
THICK, BLACK EYELINER ... CRACKED LIQUID LINER ... LINER THAT IS NOT WELL BLENDED ... LINER INSIDE YOUR LOWER LASHES ... TOO-BRIGHT EYE SHADOW ... GLITTERY EYE SHADOW ... OVERLY MATTE EYE SHADOW ... CLUMPY, HARD MASCARA ... A SINGLE LEDGE OF FALSE LASHES

happen to love the beauty business. I find most women who work in beauty to be so warm, so upbeat, so generous of spirit. I think the reason they're so happy is that they get to be around makeup all day. Makeup is our candy. All the colors, textures, brushes, pencils, pots, creams, and liquids are enough to unleash the finger-paint-loving five-year-old in all of us. This is especially true of eye makeup. The sumptuous banquet of shadow, liner, and even mascara colors is so tempting, it's tough to stay with a demure taupe when the new Easter egg shades arrive in spring or the sparkly metallics show up at holiday time. (I have limited-edition shadow compacts from Chanel and Yves Saint Laurent that I would never even place a finger on, they're so gorgeous.) So at the risk of sounding like a real killjoy, I have to tell you that once you reach a certain age, it's best to edit your makeup down to a minimalist color palette. There, I said it!

If you have bumpy eyelids, crow's-feet, or a hooded overhang, lose the thick eyeliner, the heavily pigmented colors, and the multitiered shadow effects. Instead, learn to artfully smudge a thin line of eyeliner pencil or apply a thin line of liquid liner, and stick with an understated wash of shadow in a flattering shade of beige, brown,

khaki, or gray. Wild and crazy shades of pink, purple, green, turquoise, gold, bronze, and silver shadows are only going to magnify imperfections. Shiny, glittery shadows are for kids. Thick liner, a strip of false lashes, heavily pigmented shadow, and stark white shimmer on the brow bone is the makeup of drag queens. The makeup look of the moment is soft and pretty, not hard and severe. Soft and pretty will make you look Y&H; hard and severe is so OL. "Beautiful makeup is about subtlety," says makeup artist Nick Barose, whose celebrity clients include Brooke Shields, Kim Cattrall, Sarah Jessica Parker, and Beyoncé Knowles, among others, and who has made me look younger than I ever thought possible. "When you're putting it on, step back from the mirror and make sure it looks not so noticeable."

If trendy colors aren't universally wearable, why, you might ask, do cosmetic companies create them, and why are beauty pages filled with step-by-step instructions on how to wear the hot new shades? For starters, it's tough to get buzz for your product if you're trumpeting the same tasteful brown eye shadow year after year. And how many brown shadows are you really going to buy? It takes a long time to reach the bottom of a pan of shadow. Now picture the beauty editor pitching her brown shadow idea to the editor in chief month after month: Chocolate! It's all about chocolate — again. As boring as it would be to read about the same subject issue after issue, it's even more boring to write about the same thing over and over again and try to spin it in a fresh, new direction. If you were an editor, you would welcome the chance to write about any shade that's dramatic and different. And if you were, say, twenty-three, red eye shadow might be fun on Valentine's Day. So give the red shadow and the candy-colored makeup to your daughter or your niece. Clean out your bathroom drawers and start fresh with only those products suited to a Y&H agenda.

At the top of that agenda is the modern way to do your eyes and to get you out the door with minimum fuss and maximum impact. Since I'm not a makeup artist, I've enlisted three of the best — Nick Barose, Efrat Acharkan, and Susan Sterling of Chanel — who never fail to make me look good.

The Newer Way to . . .
Do Your Eyes

Priming the Canvas
The Old Way . . . Before applying shadow, cover the top lid with foundation, then dust with loose, translucent powder.
The Newer Way . . . Before applying shadow, just smooth on a silky neutral eye primer.

Eye shadow has a habit of melting away, so we're always looking for ways to make it go on easily and stay on indefinitely. For years, makeup artists have suggested layering lids with foundation, then powder, but this takes too much time and can get messy. An eye primer is the modern solution. It's quick and easy and does double duty: it smoothes the surface for the shadow so it will stay put, and it camouflag-

es discoloration, blotchiness, and blue blood vessels and generally evens out the skin tone with a uniform palette. My favorite is Laura Mercier Eye Basics. Sometimes, when I'm in a rush, I wear Eye Basics alone and skip the shadow altogether.

Shadowing Your Eyes
The Old Way . . . Paint three distinct color blocks on the lid, one atop another, with the top tier a pearly white up to the brow bone.
The Newer Way . . . Use two neutral colors and blend them so they look natural.

Bright bands of eye shadow in deep, jewel tones are so OL: very dated, very eighties. Even if that look comes back someday (everything cycles back eventually), don't go there. It's Y&H to wear just two shadows that complement each other, as well as your eye color, hair color, and skin tone. Cover your lid in a warm, neutral shadow — "beige, taupe, off-white, or pale," says Susan Sterling, Chanel's chief international makeup artist. It should be one that is close to the color of your lid yet stands out against the color of your iris. Don't try matching your eye shadow to your eye color. "Tacky!" is the general consensus. The truth is, everyone looks good in some shade of brown, so find the best one for you. If your eyes are green, you want a brown with khaki undertones. For blue eyes, a sand or taupe color works well. Brown eyes are best shown off with a darker, almost charcoal color.

(PLEASE DON'T . . .)
Go too light on your lid (as in those dreaded opalescent whites). Aside from looking obvious, the shadow won't cover imperfections.

TOO OLD: bright bands of color and a single strip of false lashes

JUST RIGHT: blend neutral shadows and add small clusters of fake lashes

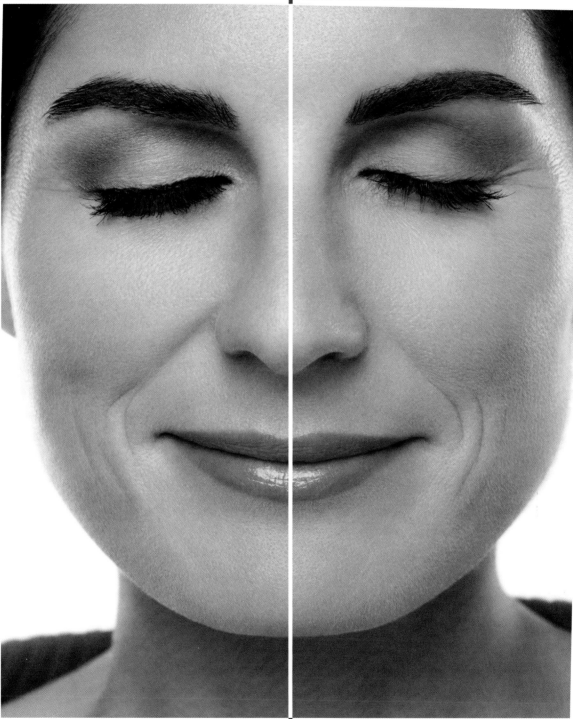

Cream or Powder Shadow?

If your lids are crepey, some cream shadows will settle into the creases faster than powders. (For excessively crepey lids, you might be better off not to put anything on them at all.) But not all powders are created equal. Stay clear of pots of loose powder that can scatter all over your face and clothes. Watch out for powders that are matte, which can appear too chalky, too dry, too OL. To make your eyes look dewy and fresh, your powder shadow should have a little luminosity — not full-on glitter, but a slight sheen. Susan Sterling recommends powder shadows with soft-focus pigments that keep them from looking flat. "When you have a subtle, luminous finish," she says, "the light bounces off and creates the illusion of a uniform, smooth surface."

For your second shadow color, choose a darker shade than your base tone. This is your definer, which goes into the crease of your eye and adds depth. To apply, dip the edge of a shadow brush into your color and follow your crease from corner to corner. With a makeup sponge or brush, blend and smudge around the edges.

Don't spend too much time searching for this color duo. Just buy the shadow kits. I like the Laura Mercier eye-color duo called Bamboo.

When you have your perfect color, dust the shadow over your entire lid, from the lash line to the brow bone, using a broad eye shadow brush. If you're low maintenance or don't want to spend much time on eye makeup, that one wash of color could be the only shadow you wear.

(PLEASE DON'T . . .)

Use your blush as eye shadow. Some makeup artists recommend that you do so in a pinch, but it will only make your eyes look bloodshot and rabbity. You're better off going without.

Where You Draw the Line

The Old Way . . . Draw a big fat line across your upper lid and rim the inside of your lower lid.
The Newer Way . . . Line the top lid close to the lashes with pencil, then smudge it to look as soft and natural as possible. Add a softly smudged, thin line under the lower lid.

"When you age, the eye area becomes less defined, so you want to line the eye, upper and lower," says Efrat, who has lined the eyes of Mariska Hargitay, Julianna Margulies, and Judi Dench. The OL way is a thick, crackled, strip of black liquid liner. The Y&H way is a thin line as close to your top lash line as possible. The goal is to look like you have a naturally dark lash line, not like you have liner on. To make the line look more organic, use a pencil (brown, forest green, or gray — black can look too harsh), then smudge it. Note to cosmetic companies: Why can't every eyeliner pencil come with a rubbery smudge tip on one end? We don't need to carry around yet another tool for smudging. (And those of us who do our makeup in the ladies' room never have a cotton swab handy!)

Luxe Lashes

The Old Way . . . Pump the brush; apply on the ends.
The Newer Way . . . Don't pump the brush; apply at the roots and brush outward.

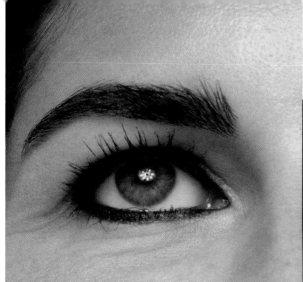

TOO OLD: thick, heavy liner

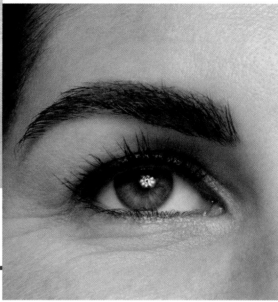

JUST RIGHT: soft and natural

LINER NOTES
What to do

✔ **When you're drawing your line,** it's more modern to start at the outer corner of the eye and draw inward, according to Nick Barose. Stop a little more than halfway. If you go the whole way in to the corner, your eye will look smaller, so use the point where your eye color ends as your stop sign.

✔ **If your lids are starting to droop,** you can try a little optical illusion. Start your line at the outer corner about a centimeter above your lashes, ever so slightly upward, then bring it down to the lash line. This will help your eye look lifted.

✔ **Try a second line** for even more drama. This is a signature technique of the great makeup artist Laura Mercier, who did this on me for a *Today* show appearance. Lift your top eyelid and line the area beneath the lashes with a dark pencil. It's a little awkward at first, but it makes your lash line look super-dark and defined without making it obvious.

✔ **Go ahead and line under the lower lid** if you don't mind drawing attention to it — that is, if you don't have puffy under-eye bags.

What not to do

✔ **Rim the inside** of your lower lash line. "Inner liner is so 1970s!" says Nick Barose. Do you remember high school, when everyone rimmed inside their lower lids with cobalt blue pencil?

✔ **Come full circle** with a thick line around your eyes, connecting the dots, so to speak, at both ends. That heavily lined eye is best left to the twenty-something Goth chicks.

✔ **Rely on retro looks.** The exaggerated cat-eye look will look OL if the tail is too long.

✔ **Trace your eyeliner** in a similar-colored shadow to make it last longer. Your liner will look unnatural and heavy. Given the choice between softness and lasting until you go to sleep, choose softness.

Pencil or Liquid Liner?

Reasonable people disagree. Nick Barose loves liquid liner because he thinks it's the best way to draw a sharp line up at the sides and defy gravity. I'd always maintained that liquid liner was too challenging in the hands of non-pros until I met Shiseido's amazingly easy-to-use Fine Eye Liner, a cartridge pen with a refill. But if you don't need that kind of precision, a sharpened pencil will do you fine. Just make sure that it has some glide. "You shouldn't have to press hard to get color. For a softer look, use a soft color like charcoal or brown," says Efrat. Makeup artist Jenna Anton, who made the models in this book look gorgeous, suggests that you buy a pencil you can sharpen (as opposed to a mechanical one) so that the tip is never dull or flat. Good point.

Luxe Lashes

Today there are dozens of mascaras designed to correct every imperfection. You can volumize, lengthen, define, curl, or fatten your lashes depending on your need. Nick Barose says that at a certain age, you want length, not volume; longer but not fiber-y. "High volume will give you chunky lashes that will age you," he says. Makeup pros favor a small, thin wand over a big fat one. The not-so-dirty little secret is that there are awesome mascaras at every price point. The key to creating the most flattering, fluttering frame of lashes is application.

Efrat swears that when she applies mascara to her clients' lashes, they look four times bigger than when the clients do it themselves.

I believe her, because I've seen it. So what are we doing wrong? First, don't pump. We've all gotten in the habit of pumping our mascara several times to remove excess on the brush. Moving the wand in and out of the tube draws air into it, drying out the mascara and making it thick and sticky, which increases the likelihood of clumps. Second, to get the fullest, lushest lashes possible, start the stroke at the base of the roots, never the middle or ends, and wiggle the brush around a little. Then draw the brush out to the tips. This way, your lashes will look as long as possible, and even after you apply three or four coats, they won't stick together in brittle, Tammy Faye–like clumps. "Mascara gives you

JUST RIGHT: Angela Bassett's subtly sexy eyes

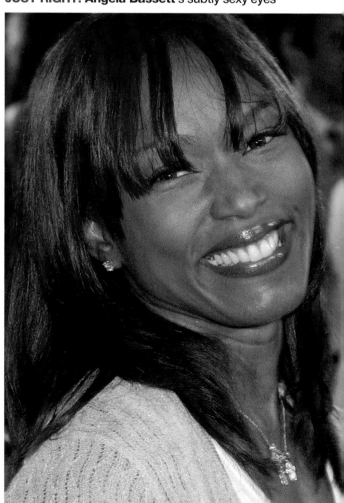

Extra Eye To-Dos

✔ **Invest in a Good Magnifying Mirror with a Light**
"Don't hesitate to use it when applying liner, because your eyesight isn't what it was in your twenties," says Efrat.

✔ **Whiten Up**
When you age, the whites of your eyes may not look as bright as they once did, so use eyedrops to banish the red. The bloodshot and bleary-eyed look is OL.

a youthful look; it makes you look awake," says Efrat, who loves her Yves Saint Laurent magic wand and believes you can get away with "just wearing mascara all day and no other eye make-up. . . . After you've put it all over, go from the inside out and push the lashes a little upward." The bottom lashes are not as important as the top, but she thinks that you need to do them to get a nice frame for the entire eye.

As with eyeliner, don't go crazy with color. Magenta, purple, and green are really more about theater. Stick with basic black unless you have very light hair and a light complexion. If black looks too hard, try dark brown.

Before putting on mascara, use an eyelash curler to help open up your eyes, even if you're about to use curling mascara. (Why not get all the curl you can?) Efrat raves about the Shu Ue-mura curler because it doesn't pinch and won't break your lashes. You may have wondered about heated eyelash curlers or using a hair dryer to heat one up. Bad idea. It's dangerous to use heat that close to the sensitive eye area.

Another option is lash tinting, a more permanent solution that involves having your lashes tinted black or brown at a salon. Tinting can be irritating to the eye, and there's always the risk of your lashes falling out. The more modern way to achieve dark, lush lashes is lash extensions or growing your own with a "miracle grow" lash product (read on).

FAKING IT WITH FALSIES
The Old Way . . . Apply a single strip of lashes across your entire lash line.
The Newer Way . . . Apply a few small clusters of fake lashes.

If you're going out for the evening and really want to ramp up the glamour quotient, add a few extra lashes. Avoid a full ledge of lashes — too fake, too OL. It's easy to find tiny clusters of fake lashes at drugstores, beauty supply shops, and makeup emporiums such as Sephora. Each cluster holds about eight hairs. Using a tweezer, dip the tip of a cluster into eyelash glue and stick it in between your own lashes, wherever you have a gap. Don't forget to add a few at the outer corners of your eyes. Five clusters per eye should be more than enough. Then brush on mascara so your own lashes and your new ones blend together. Bat your lashes — and smile!

Drastic Measures for Lost Eyelashes, Droopy Lids, and Under-Eye Bags

Women who have lost their eyelashes due to injury or illness can have an eyelash transplant. Hair from your scalp is sewn onto your lids, hair by hair, and then grows in like the hair on your head (not like lash hair), so it needs to be curled, cut, and possibly dyed. This is extremely high maintenance, but as more and more women lose lashes to chemotherapy, this surgery is gaining in popularity, according to hair transplant specialist Dr. Alan Bauman. He is based in Boca Raton, Florida, and charges $3,000 per eye.

If your upper lids are drooping and hooded, if your lower lids have bulging fat deposits or permanent puffiness, or if your eyes look irreparably old and tired, there is only so much magic makeup can do. Granted, some women — Lauren Bacall, Charlotte Rampling — have made a career out of sexy, hooded eyelids, but not me. A few years ago, when my upper eyelids started sagging, I went to a plastic surgeon for a blepharoplasty. In this procedure, also known as an eyelid plasty, the surgeon removes excess skin and fat from your upper or lower lids. (I only had my upper lids done, but it's common to have fatty under-eye bags removed, too.) It was one of the best beauty decisions I've ever made. The surgery lasted about an hour, and I was back at work in a week. Sometimes, when the upper lids get really saggy, they can impair vision, and this surgery becomes a necessity.

I never let mine get to that point and because it was never "that bad," no one ever knew. Until now.

$ Is It Worth It?

Lash Extensions. Women looking for longer-lasting, lush lashes can have lash extensions applied at a salon. It's a two-hour process that should last three months. A lash pro will bond fifty to sixty individual lashes, lash by lash, to your own lashes, and afterward you will have such long, luxe lashes that no mascara is needed. I did a *Today* show segment on lash extensions, and the results were amazing. Upside: Women who have very thin, sparse lashes and aren't satisfied with the results they get from mascara may find lash extensions well worth the $300 price tag. Downside: Lashes do fall off, and you'll need to get "filled" every two to three weeks ($85 or so a filling).

GROWING YOUR OWN LASHES LONGER

Age Intervention Eyelash Conditioner by Jan Marini Skin Research is a newer and lower-maintenance way to achieve long, lush lashes. Although the conditioner is not inexpensive ($160), you just apply it with a mascara-like wand to your own lash line. Wexler Dermatology sells it because of the results seen on patients. If you use this product, you might have to start trimming your lashes!

EYE PRIMER
Laura Mercier Eye Basics, $22; Saks, 877-551-7257; lauramercier.com

EYE SHADOW
Clé de Peau Beauté Eye Color Quad, $70; Saks, 877-551-7257; Neiman Marcus, 888-888-4757
Christian Dior 5-Colour Eyeshadow, $52; Sephora, 877-737-4672 or sephora.com
NARS Single Eye Shadow in Lola Lola, $21; Sephora, 877-737-4672 or sephora.com; narscosmetics.com
Laura Mercier Evolution of Colour for Eyes in Brown Velvet, $36; Saks, 877-551-7257; lauramercier.com
Laura Mercier Eye Colour Duo in Bamboo, $22; Neiman Marcus, 888-888-4757; lauramercier.com
Laura Mercier Eye Colour in Vanilla Nuts, $20; Saks, 877-551-7257; lauramercier.com
Revlon ColorStay 12 Hour Eye Shadow Quad in Coffee Bean, $6.99; drugstores and mass retailers

EYELINER
Christian Dior Crayon Eyeliner Pencil, $24; Sephora, 877-737-4672 or sephora.com
Prescriptives Softlining Pencil, $17.50; Bloomingdale's, 800-555-7467; prescriptives.com
Revlon ColorStay Eyeliner, $7.39, drugstores and mass retailers
Shiseido The Makeup Fine Eye Liner, $27; Macy's, 800-289-6229 or macys.com
Styli-Style Liquid Liner 24, $8; styli-style.com

EYELASH CURLER
Shu Uemura Eyelash Curler, $18; Shu Uemura, 888-748-5678 or shuuemura-usa.com

MASCARA
Lancôme Hypnôse Custom Volume Mascara, $23; Saks, 877-551-7257; lancome.com
Clinique High Definition Lashes, $13.50; Bloomingdale's, 800-555-7467; clinique.com
CoverGirl VolumeExact Mascara, $6.99; drugstores and mass retailers

Maybelline New York Define-A-Lash Mascara, $7.49; drugstores and mass retailers
Yves Saint Laurent Everlong Lengthening Mascara, $26.50; Saks, 877-551-7257; Nordstrom, nordstrom.com

EYE MAKEUP REMOVER
Almay Non-Oily Eye Makeup Remover Pads, $4.99; drugstores and mass retailers
Clarins Gentle Eye Make-Up Remover Lotion, $24; clarins.com

FAUX LASHES
Make Up For Ever Individual Faux Lashes, $14; Sephora, 877-737-4672 or sephora.com
Shu Uemura Flare Eyelashes, $15; Shu Uemura, 888-748-5678 or shuuemura-usa.com

LASH LENGTHENING
Jan Marini Age Intervention Eyelash Conditioner, $160; dermastore.com

LOSE THE HEAVY EYELINER

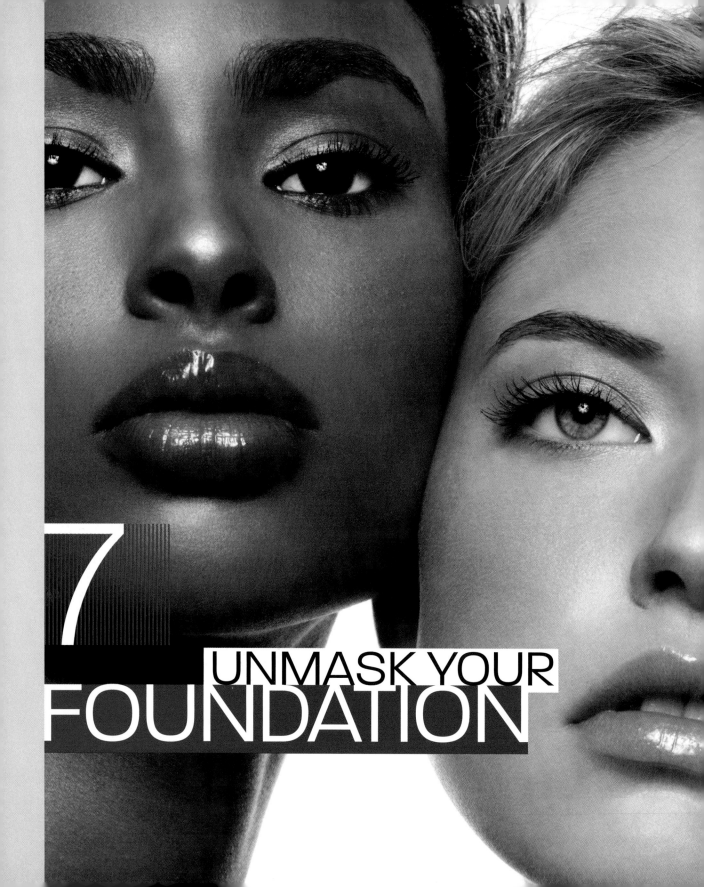

7

UNMASK YOUR FOUNDATION

NOTHING AGES YOU LIKE...
FOUNDATION THAT IS TOO THICK, TOO CAKEY, OR OVERLY MATTE... A DEMARCATION LINE BETWEEN YOUR CHIN AND NECK... RACCOON EYES... STREAKS OF BLUSH... ASHY FACE POWDER... LOOKING TOO TAN

One of the headlines in the tabloids that always makes me smile while I'm standing in the supermarket checkout is "Stars Without Makeup." If you thumb through the pages, you'll see all the proof you need that not even Nicole Kidman looks like the Nicole Kidman we see on magazine covers without going through the glamour assembly line — hair colorist, hairdresser, makeup artist, stylist, manicurist — and then to the retoucher, where her image is tweaked to perfection. If you have any doubt that you, too, would look gorgeous given all that help, you need only look at the groundbreaking Dove video *Evolution,* released on the company's Web site in the fall of 2006. The video shows an everyday-looking woman transformed into a beauty superstar courtesy of the glamour assembly line and hundreds of hours of photo retouching. Like everything else in our culture, beauty has been hyped up, and we've fallen in love with an unreal, idealized version of how we're supposed to look. There's hardly a beauty photo in a magazine editorial, ad, or book that hasn't been retouched, and we're so used to seeing "unreal" beauty that we don't know what real beauty looks like. Which brings me to an interesting paradox: all the beauty work I talk about in this book is to look as if you've done nothing. The Y&H look is radiant beauty, glowing skin, and looking like you are not wearing makeup. In this chapter, I'll teach you how to use more product than ever so that you can look as if you're not wearing any makeup at all!

"People on the street now look like they have good skin, and you don't know whether they're wearing foundation or not," says makeup pro Nick Barose. "That's good foundation. We all want to look like we have beautiful skin." And it's easier than ever to look like you do (even if you don't) thanks to new products made with silicone, a new age Vaseline-like substance that makes the best primers, foundations, concealers, and lip products glide on seamlessly. My friend Lois Joy Johnson, beauty and fashion director of *More* magazine, jokes about silicone. "Don't leave home without it!" Products made with silicone help fill in lines and smooth skin so that the surface feels like silk, and you need much less to do the trick. Foundations themselves also are improving constantly, so now you can get the coverage you need without looking like a geisha. The latest foundations contain light-reflecting luminizers and are so technologically advanced that they manage to do the Triple Lutz: they are transparent enough to look natural, provide good coverage, and blend into any skin color. This is true for foundations in every price range.

So if you're wearing an OL mask of foundation, the first thing you need to do is lighten up. Take advantage of these new products that use state-of-the-art science to help us fill in the cracks and look like we have light radiating out of our pores. In other words, they help us look perfect — as perfect as possible without retouching.

BE YOUR OWN BEAUTY EDITOR

If there is a downside to these technological breakthroughs, it is the massive amount of products we have to choose from. We can't fit them *all* into our tiny cosmetic bags. To edit down all your choices and find what's truly best for you, you have to become your own beauty editor. Of course, you've been editing your beauty choices forever. I'm just going to give you a methodical way to do it. After all, no one went to school to study beauty editing. Beauty editors are people who love to play with products and test them out. This book is filled with products that work for me. Only by putting them on your face can you determine whether they work for you.

So let's test foundations. After you gather up all the foundations worth trying, test two at a time by applying one product to one half of your face and the second product to the other half of your face. In this face-off, you can usually tell immediately which side looks more radiant, which foundation glides on more easily, and which one feels more comfortable. Next, wash your face and test the winner of the first round with the next contender. Continue the process until you've tested all the foundations. (You might want to stretch this out over a few days!) At the end of this exercise, you will know what's best for you. This is the best way to test every beauty product, from foundations to primers to mascaras to blush. I often walk out of the house with two different brands on my face. To record your research, keep a little beauty journal with a pen in a bathroom drawer. When you go out shopping, throw the journal in your bag so there's no guessing about the exact shade and formulation you want to buy.

Obviously, this research can get very expensive if you're not getting free products from the beauty companies, so ask for samples. Sephora is very generous and will let you sample almost anything. And did you know that you can return almost any makeup product purchased at a department store? The makeup companies are going to kill me for saying this, but as long as you don't try to return, say, a half-empty bottle six months after you bought it, they will probably take it back. Many drugstores, too, have a more liberal return policy than you might expect, taking back makeup if it is the wrong shade, even if you've opened it. Rite Aid guarantees this with a receipt. (Call your local drugstore to check on its policy.) If you've bought a product you don't like but can't be bothered to return it, toss it into a plastic "reject bin." Maybe a shade that doesn't work for you will work for your mother, your sister, or a friend. My nieces are probably the only girls in Buffalo Grove, Illinois, who have been painting their fingernails and toenails with Chanel polish since kindergarten! Unopened makeup is also a welcome donation at women's organizations such as Bottomless Closet.

CREATING THE PERFECT CANVAS

There are not many problems that makeup can't cover. If your complexion is blotchy or blemished; has red patches, brown age spots, blue veins, or purple under-eye circles; or is freckled or flaky, the right makeup can smooth it out and create the perfect canvas. The opportunity to look as if you have naturally flawless skin is within your reach, especially now that products are so advanced and easy to use.

If you are fortunate enough to possess flawless skin and your problem is just uneven color, you can get away with wearing just a tinted moisturizer. All the major companies make one. The gold standard, the one that consistently wins "best of" in this category, is Laura Mercier Tinted Moisturizer with SPF 20. If you don't have flawless skin, you might want to add it to your beauty arsenal for weekends or the gym. When you need

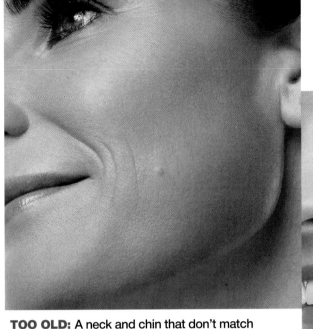

TOO OLD: A neck and chin that don't match

more ammunition, use the latest weapons the beauty counter has to offer to put your best Y&H face forward.

Covering Your Bases: Foundation
The OL Way . . .
Foundation Applied Like Paint over the Entire Face

How do you know if you're using the wrong foundation? If you're using a lot of it and your skin looks as if it needs to be excavated from under layers of makeup, it's time to buy a new one. "Don't think of covering up all the imperfections," warns Nick Barose. "Remember, you are not painting a wall." Not only do thick foundations look OL, but they are holdovers from the cosmetic dark ages. Even though the newer foundations are lighter, they don't skimp on coverage.

The Y&H Way . . .
Foundation Applied Sparingly over Primer

When I was testing out all my Brilliant Buys with a few friends, I discovered that not one of them used primer. If you're not currently using primer, stop reading, pick up the phone, and order this one now: Smashbox Photo Finish Foundation Primer SPF 15 with Dermaxyl Complex, $42; Sephora,

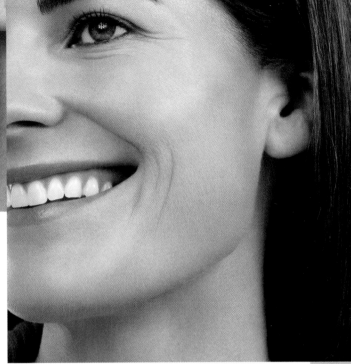

JUST RIGHT: Is she even wearing foundation?

877-737-4672 or smashbox.com. I don't mean to be overly dramatic, but what if they sell out? What if they stop making it? Every one of my testers e-mailed me the next day asking where they could buy this primer. Unless your skin is flawless, you need primer under your foundation. Today there is a burgeoning beauty category of products designed to prep the skin for foundation, and primer is a star product in this category.

As you can probably guess by the name, face primer acts just like paint primer, readying and evening out the "canvas." The main ingredient in most primers is silicone. Silicone, that truly miraculous, invisible gel that we spoke of earlier, makes skin feel soft but not sticky. It smoothes over wrinkles and pores so that makeup doesn't settle into

The newer foundations are so smart that they adapt to your skin tone.

them, tightens skin, and fills in fine lines. It makes skin smooth as glass so that foundation glides on. It also gives your foundation something to adhere to, so it lasts longer and doesn't get splotchy. You apply the primer all over the face after moisturizer and before foundation.

One caveat: Some primers can be drying. Nick Barose suggests testing one on the back of your hand and seeing how it performs. If it gets flaky or settles noticeably into creases, it's not the one for you.

The Newer Way to . . .

Apply Foundation

The days of just slapping on moisturizer and then foundation are over. Now there are many more steps to achieve great-looking skin, but the results are definitely worth the effort.

1. **Cleanse.**
2. **Exfoliate (see chapter 8).**
3. **Restore (with a serum).**
4. **Moisturize (with sunscreen).**
5. **Prime.**
6. **Apply foundation.**

Priming the skin can include more than foundation primers. Now, if you walk into Sephora or any department store, you will see a whole host of products for skin prep. There are wrinkle-erasing products, skin brighteners, light reflectors, light diffusers, luminizers, and skin perfectors. No

matter what they call themselves, these products either deflect light, which helps diffuse the look of fine lines, or add luminosity, which we know is important as we get older and our skin starts to lose its natural dewiness. Go ahead and test these out to see which ones work best for you. If you don't have time to add these to your daily makeup routine, I hear you. For special events, I use Clarins Instant Light Complexion Perfector, a light reflector that also adds luminosity, layered over Clarins Instant Smooth Perfecting Touch Primer (which deflects wrinkles). The makeup artist Efrat, whom I introduced in chapter 6, is a master at prepping the skin so that it glows. In a makeup hour, I'd say that her skin prep takes forty-five minutes and applying the actual makeup fifteen minutes. Most of these products are transparent, so you can layer them on top of one another. Some foundations also include a luminizer so make sure you read the package and don't buy something you already have.

As any dermatologist will tell you, one of your face products must include a sunscreen with at least SPF 30. I think it's best to get your SPF in your moisturizer (Dr. Pat Wexler's moisturizers all have SPF 30, see Brilliant Buys in the next chapter). But you can also get it in, say, your foundation. (See more on avoiding the sun later in this chapter.)

Getting It On: Applying Foundation

The point of using primer is to make your skin look so great that you need less foundation, which is one reason I prefer putting my foundation on with my fingers. If my skin is looking good one morning, I can just dab base on the places I need it and blend it in. Personally, I think foundation brushes are impractical. For one thing, I have yet to figure out how to achieve the same kind of control I get using my fingers. More pragmatically, if you don't clean the brush every day, the bristles will be matted and cakey the next time you use it. Who wants to wash a makeup brush every day? I'd much rather wash my hands. As for sponges, you end up wasting a lot of product. Sponges also get kind of gross quickly, so you have to buy a new one every two weeks, which is high maintenance.

The OL Way . . .
The Matte Look
When you were young, chances are your biggest problem was oily skin and acne, so you chose an oil-free foundation to cut down on shine and breakouts. Most mature skin is drier, so oil-free formulas have a tendency to look matte and chalky (unless you still have oily skin). You want your skin to look luminous, not flat. Another problem with the matte look is that it appears too "done," as if you have just left a session with your makeup artist. So OL!

The Y&H Way . . .
The Dewy Look
It's time to get over your fear of oil. Since most women our age need moisture and hydration, we also need a creamy foundation. If you have truly oily skin that hasn't changed since you were a teenager or you are having a bout of adult acne, go ahead and choose an oil-free foundation. But if you have normal or dry skin, a hydrating foundation will not only make your skin look refreshed and moisturized, but it also will help plump up lines so they are less visible. Love that.

(PLEASE DON'T . . .)
Slather foundation all over your neck. Yes, it's admirable to try to avoid having a division between your chin and your neck, but this is not the way to achieve harmony. You want to treat your neck as well as you treat your face when it comes to cleansing, exfoliating, and moisturizing. This will help prevent it from getting too jowly and lined. But don't take things any further. For daytime, smooth foundation just below your jawline and blend. If you spread it too far down your neck, it will come off on your collar, which is about as good a look as lipstick on your teeth. So OL! If, for a special occasion, you are wearing a top that's low-cut or plunging, you can add tinted moisturizer farther down your neck and on your décolletage, but do it sparingly and dust it with translucent powder to help set it.

True Colors: Your Makeup Match
It used to be a nightmare to find your color match in foundation, especially in a drugstore, where you can't sample and have to rely instead on laminated plastic swatches that bear no resemblance to human skin. Now women don't need to worry as much about finding an exact match, because the newer foundations are so smart that they adapt to your skin tone. I know I sound as if I drank the Kool-Aid, but I saw a demo for CoverGirl TruBlend Foundation that made me a believer. In a room of jaded beauty editors, an African American woman and a Caucasian woman chose the same middle-level shade from about fifteen shades. Both women applied the foundation in front of us and then walked around so that we could see them close-up. Both looked as if they had found their foundation soul mate! CoverGirl is so confident about its TruBlend line that it offers a money-back guarantee if the shade you buy doesn't turn out to be a perfect match. L'Oréal Paris has its version, the award-winning True Match. Because matchability isn't the problem that it once was, Nick Barose says that

when he goes out on a job, he doesn't have to bring as many shades of foundation as he used to. This is especially welcome news for women with darker skin tones, who have always had difficulty finding mainstream brands with the right color range. (FYI: Revlon, Clinique, Bobbi Brown, MAC, and Prescriptives offer a wide range.)

The newer way to try on foundation in a department store is to test it directly on your jawline, not your hand. Then walk outside into the daylight and look in a mirror. If you can't see where the foundation starts and ends on your skin, it's a match. If you're in doubt or you're between two colors, go with the lighter shade. It's better for skin to look slightly brighter than darker. You may want to buy both shades and use the lighter one in the winter and the darker one in the summer.

Don't want to deal with this matching issue? You don't have to. Go to a Prescriptives counter near you that offers Custom Blend Foundation. (Not every department store features this, but 185 do. Go to prescriptives.com to find one near you.) The makeup pro will "color print" you on the spot and whip up a batch of foundation to perfectly match your skin. By the way, I don't know what I would do without the travel-size bottle of foundation that Prescriptives gives you in addition to the full-size one . . . It's the only foundation bottle I've found that is small enough to toss directly into my makeup bag. Why more companies don't offer travel-size foundation, I have no idea.

The Great Cover-Up: Concealer
The OL Way . . .
Concealer That Is Too Cakey, Too Thick, Too Light, or Too Obvious
Every woman who is sleep deprived and overworked (in other words, everyone) loves a good concealer. But if it's too pasty, too white, or too bright, you get the dreaded raccoon look, which can accentuate wrinkles and crepey skin. You

never want to create a solution that's worse than the problem.

The Y&H Way . . .
Concealer That Melts into Skin
If you could use only one beauty product, what would it be? For me, it would be concealer. More specifically, Clé de Peau Beauté. At $68, it's a splurge, but it lasts a good two years and can be used, in a pinch, as foundation or eye shadow or to cover age spots, wrinkles, or zits. Use concealer after foundation; you'll use less. You want a concealer that's creamy, not runny. You should be able to rub it between your fingers and watch it melt into your skin.

What color concealer? Consider the color of the circles you want to cover. Susan Sterling says that if the area under your eyes looks brownish or purple, choose a concealer with a touch of yellow. If the shadows are gray, use a concealer that's more beige and rosy. And to further diminish the appearance of lines, look for a concealer that has some light-reflecting pigments (read the package).

A Touch of Pink
The OL Way . . .
Using Blush for Contouring
A lot of women our age have trouble with blush. Whether it's color or application, it just doesn't look natural. Forget trying to resculpt the look of your face with blush. You've no doubt seen the articles in beauty magazines that suggest you can create jutting cheekbones with a pan of blush or contouring powder. Even if you could master the technique like a pro, Nick Barose points out, it's a trick best done by a makeup artist on a model in a situation where the photographer can control the light and the result is a two-dimensional image. Otherwise, it looks phony, because, as Nick points

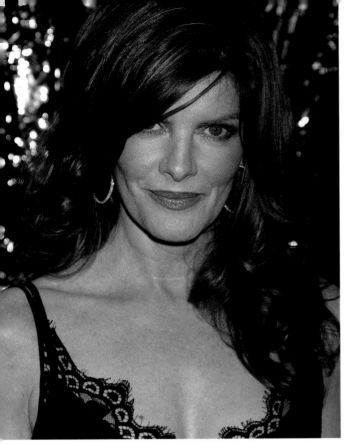

JUST RIGHT: Rene Russo's Y&H complexion perfection

out, "in real life people are seeing you at different angles." Women who attempt to contour usually end up with two pink streaks down the sides of their cheeks in the shape of the Nike symbol. It's one of those things that can make you look so OL — and a little batty.

The Y&H Way . . .
Using Blush to Look Like You're Blushing
A natural-looking blush will instantly make you look younger and fresher, like you just came in from jogging or had great sex (which is why NARS named one of the best blushes of all time Orgasm). One of the easier things you can do to look Y&H is to switch from powder to cream blush. (I love NARS Orgasm, which is a powder, but I love NARS Penny Lane, a cream blush, even more.) What a difference this tiny change can make! One caveat: Cream blush tends to fade quickly, so there is a trade-off. But come on! Wouldn't you prefer to

touch up a Y&H face than to have an OL face that is longer lasting?

What color blush? Stay away from anything too dark. If you have fair skin, go with a pale, rosy pink. For medium skin, choose a blush that's more coral or peachy. If you have darker skin, try a brownish orange, such as mango. Don't be scared off by the brightness; after you've blended it in, it will give you just the right amount of pop. You can always try matching your blush to your lipstick. Efrat suggests taking your favorite lipstick to a makeup counter and asking for a blush in the same color family.

Sponge or fingers? Nick Barose advises using a sponge for this job; I prefer to use my fingers. After foundation, put a dot of creamy blush on the apple of each cheek, then blend up and out so there are no obvious edges.

The Finishing Touch: Powder
The OL Way . . .
A Matte Finish via Dry, Chalky Powder
On an *Oprah* show about aging, TV's Diane Sawyer declared powder "the enemy" of old age. She's right: a dusting of chalky powder will settle into fine lines, deaden your glow, and leave you with a nasty residue of ashiness.

The Y&H Way . . .
A Luminous Finish via Silky, Translucent Powder
But there's a new generation of powders that are feathery light and completely translucent and that leave you with a luminous sheen. Look for powders that are light-reflecting or light-diffusing to obscure fine lines or imperfections. If you can sample the powder, rub a little between your fingers. It should feel moist and silky, not grainy. Makeup artist

Jenna Anton and I both love Laura Mercier Secret Brightening Powder. Efrat is a fan of powders from Chanel and Givenchy. At the drugstore, try L'Oréal Paris Translucide Naturally Luminous Powder. After applying foundation, concealer, and blush, dip your brush into the powder, tap any excess off into the sink, and lightly dust your face. Powder helps cut down on oily shine and sets your makeup, preventing it from melting off.

Don't attempt to carry loose powder around with you. Even if you transfer it into a tiny plastic container, you're going to have a mess on your hands or clothes. For on-the-go touch-ups, use a pressed powder compact (see Brilliant Buys).

THE ANTI-BRONZE AGE

If your skin is a little leathery, a little too wrinkled and weathered, it's probably because we are the last generation of women to grow up oblivious to the dangers of tanning. Can you believe that we once covered record albums with aluminum foil and poured homemade solutions of baby oil and iodine on our bodies to better catch the rays? To repent for all that damage, we have no choice but to slather on sunscreen with at least SPF 30 on our faces (and at least SPF 15 on any other exposed body part) even on cloudy days. If you can't give up the sun completely, limit your exposure between the hours of 11:00 a.m. and 2:00 p.m., when the sun is the strongest, plus wear a hat and sunglasses. You already know all this, but it can't be said often enough. Aside from the fact that exposure to UV rays can kill, the lizard-lady permatan is so OL and phony-looking. "Pale is beautiful" role models include Nicole Kidman, Madonna, Cate Blanchett, Julianne Moore, and Gwen Stefani — women who look as if they never hit the beach. A bronze face is gorgeous on a woman who is naturally bronze (such as Jennifer Lopez) and is just enhancing her skin glow. In other words, to be Y&H is be true to the skin you're in.

In the summer, however, there's no tan like a faux tan. If you must get rid of the pasty look, use a self-tanner or bronzer on your face, but err on the side of subtle. You want your face, neck, and arms to be all the same color. For details on self-tanning, see chapter 17.

(PLEASE DON'T . . .)

Go near a tanning booth. There are much more modern, healthier ways to get your glow.

BRILLIANT BUYS

CONCEALER
Benefit Boi-ing Industrial Strength Concealer, $20; Macy's, 800-289-6229; Benefit Cosmetics, benefitcosmetics.com
Clé de Peau Beauté Concealer, $68; Saks, 877-551-7257; Neiman Marcus, 888-888-4757
YSL Touche Éclat Radiant Touch, $39.50; Saks, 877-551-7257; Nordstrom, nordstrom.com

TINTED MOISTURIZER
Laura Mercier Tinted Moisturizer SPF 20, $40; Neiman Marcus, 888-888-4757; Laura Mercier, lauramercier.com
For non-tinted moisturizers, see the next chapter.

LUMINIZERS
Clarins Instant Light Complexion Perfector, $28; Clarins, clarins.com
MAC Strobe Cream, $29.50; MAC, 800-387-6707 or maccosmetics.com

FOUNDATION PRIMER
Senna Cosmetics Silky Primer, $36; Senna Cosmetics, 800-537-3662 or sennacosmetics.com
Smashbox Photo Finish Foundation Primer SPF 15 with Dermaxyl Complex, $42; Sephora, 877-737-4672 or sephora.com; Smashbox Cosmetics, smashbox.com

FOUNDATION

Chantecaille Future Skin Foundation, $65; Neiman Marcus, 888-888-4757 or neimanmarcus.com

Chantecaille Real Skin SPF 30 Foundation in Glow, $62; Neiman Marcus, 888-888-4757 or neimanmarcus.com

Clarins True Radiance Foundation, $36; Clarins, clarins.com

CoverGirl Advanced Radiance Restorative Cream Foundation, $9.99; drugstores and mass retailers

CoverGirl TruBlend Whipped Foundation, $7.99; drugstores and mass retailers

Laura Mercier Moisturizing Foundation, $40; Saks, 877-551-7257; Laura Mercier, lauramercier.com

L'Oréal Paris Age Perfect Skin-Support & Hydrating Makeup, $16.59; drugstores and mass retailers

L'Oréal Paris True Match Super-Blendable Makeup, $9.99; drugstores and mass retailers

Prescriptives Custom Blend Foundation, $62; Prescriptives, prescriptives.com

Prescriptives Flawless Skin Total Protection Makeup SPF 15, $39.50; Prescriptives, prescriptives.com

Revlon Age Defying Makeup and Concealer Compact, $13.99; drugstores and mass retailers

OIL-FREE FOUNDATION

Prescriptives Virtual Skin Super-Natural Finish, $32.50; Prescriptives, prescriptives.com

LOOSE POWDER

Laura Mercier Loose Setting Powder in Translucent, $32; Saks, 877-551-7257; Laura Mercier, lauramercier.com

Laura Mercier Secret Brightening Powder, $22; Neiman Marcus, 888-888-4757; lauramercier.com

L'Oréal Paris Translucide Naturally Luminous Powder, $10.75; drugstores and mass retailers

Shiseido The Makeup Enriched Loose Powder, $32; Macy's, 800-289-6229 or macys.com

POWDER COMPACT

CoverGirl Advanced Radiance Age-Defying Compact Makeup, $9.99; drugstores and mass retailers

Lancôme Dual Finish Versatile Powder Makeup, $34.50; Saks, 877-551-7257; Lancôme, lancome.com

MAC Blot Powder, $20; MAC, 800-387-6707 or maccosmetics.com

NARS Pressed Powder in Eden, $28; Sephora, 877-737-4672 or sephora.com; NARS, narscosmetics.com

Sally Hansen CornSilk Shineless Classic Translucent Pressed Powder, $5.49; drugstores and mass retailers

T. LeClerc Pressed Powder in Sable, $46; Barneys, barneys.com

BLUSH

L'Oréal Paris HIP High Intensity Pigments Blendable Blushing Créme, $10; drugstores and mass retailers

NARS Blush in Orgasm, $25; Sephora, 877-737-4672 or sephora.com; NARS, narscosmetics.com

NARS Creme Blush in Penny Lane, $23; Sephora, 877-737-4672 or sephora.com; NARS, narscosmetics.com

Paula Dorf Cheek Color Cream, $19; Sephora, 877-737-4672 or sephora.com

BRONZER

YSL Sun Powder SPF 10, $44; Saks, 877-551-7257; Nordstrom, nordstrom.com

MAKEUP BRUSHES

Clinique Brush Collection, $10.50–$32.50; Bloomingdale's, 800-555-7467; Clinique, clinique.com

Kevyn Aucoin Large Blush & Powder Brush, $65; Kevyn Aucoin, kevynaucoin.com

Kevyn Aucoin The Brush Collection, $350; Kevyn Aucoin, kevynaucoin.com

Mark Brushes, $5–$8; Mark, meetmark.com

Sonia Kashuk Deluxe Brush Set, $19.99; Target, target.com

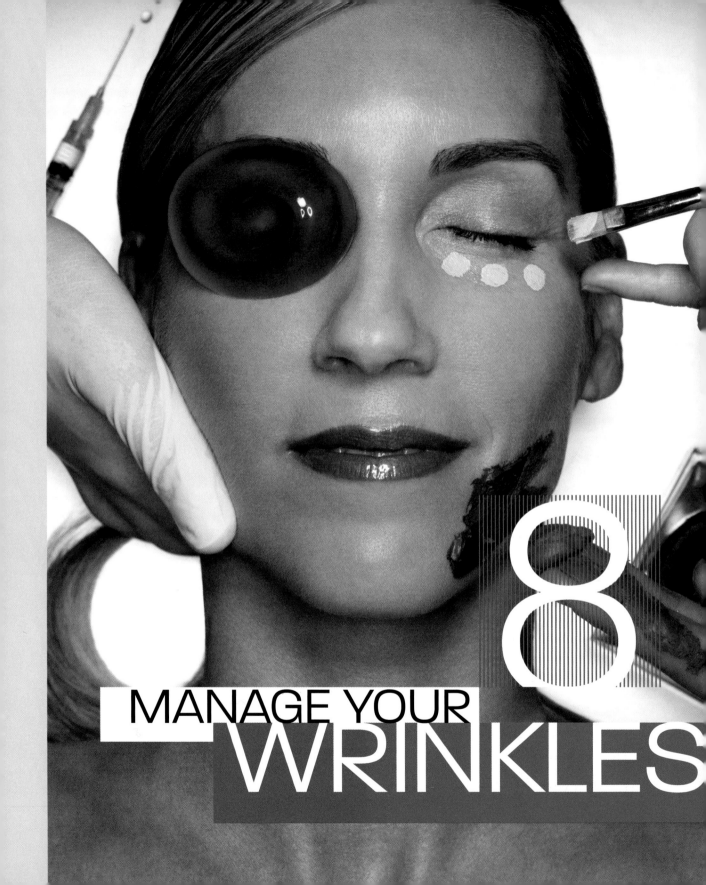

8
MANAGE YOUR WRINKLES

NOTHING AGES YOU LIKE . . .
FOREHEAD LINES . . . CROW'S-FEET . . . LIP LINES . . . SMILE LINES . . . MARIONETTE LINES . . . SAGGING SKIN . . . AGE SPOTS . . . DRY SKIN

This whole book is based on the idea of fast and easy fixes to make you look Y&H, whether you are looking for high-, medium-, or low-maintenance solutions. But I'm going to be honest with you: when it comes to making wrinkles disappear, the fastest fixes can be found at your dermatologist's office. There is no fast fix in a jar of cream at the drugstore (yet) that can make wrinkles disappear before your eyes. And anything done at the doctor's office — from a vast menu of injectable fillers and freezers to peels and lasers — is going to be expensive. But visiting a doctor is the only way we have right now to see real results short of plastic surgery (which is neither fast nor easy).

What do I mean by "real results"? I mean a difference you can clearly see when you look in the mirror. When cosmetic companies tout the results of their products, they're often talking about a change visible if you looked at your skin under a microscope. Who does that? A topical cream — even an expensive one — is not going to give you that "Wow, what a difference!" reaction when you check yourself out in the mirror. But getting an injection of Botox or a wrinkle filler *will* give you that result, if not right there on the spot, then a few days later.

First, though, let's talk about what the dermatologist can do for you. I'm a big fan of injectables, because I've seen the results on my own face. I think they're the best thing we have in our antiaging arsenal. I've had Botox injections to smooth the furrows in my forehead and my crow's-feet. I've had Restylane, CosmoPlast, and CosmoDerm injections to fill smile and marionette lines, and I know they can work wonders. I personally haven't done much with lasers. I had a couple of sessions with the Fraxel laser that did result in some improvements in my skin texture and tone, but I didn't have the patience to complete the six-session series. So for me, the jury is still out on whether laser treatments are worth the price and the pain.

Yes, pain. It hurts to be beautiful! You have to tell yourself things like that, because if you have a low threshold for pain, you will find that these injections and lasers *kill.* And the redness and inflammation that occur afterward are not to be minimized. Drug companies advertise these minimally invasive procedures as "lunchtime" treatments, but don't think for a second that they are easy, breezy no-big-deals. Let's just say that it's best not to make plans afterward. Better to schedule your appointment after work or on a day off so you can go home to recover. Even if you have just a few minor red spots and needle pricks, who wants to go back to the office looking like that? In her book *Beauty Junkies,* Alex Kuczynski offers a cautionary tale of her own Restylane injections gone terribly wrong — in the hands of a top-notch doctor she trusted. You never know how your skin will react to a particular procedure, even if it's not the first time around.

So if you can deal with the pain and the expense, these nonsurgical solutions are your best options for getting rid of a shopping list of aging

Be very wary of anyone offering cheap injections. A cut-rate price on set-price brands such as Botox or Restylane should raise a serious red flag. Botox comes as a cold powder that is diluted with saline before being injected. Doctors who offer discount prices on Botox injections are most likely diluting it more to make it go further. But the more diluted the Botox, the less time your results will last. That "bargain" injection will wear off quickly and send you back to the doctor for more. That's no bargain! Dr. Gerstner has a suggestion for less expensive full-potency injections: see if a local teaching hospital offers discounted treatments administered by a resident. Your call.

woes — wrinkles, brown spots, sagging skin, and more. Smart shoppers should know that the list of options at the dermatologist's office keeps changing. New fillers are being approved by the Food and Drug Administration (FDA) every year, and new lasers and other skin-enhancing gizmos are relentlessly touted as the Next Big Thing. Just FYI, doctors tend to be partial to one solution over another. So one might suggest filling your marionette lines with one filler, another might suggest something different, a third might suggest a combination of the two (called layering), and a fourth might tell you that you need a filler plus a laser to see any significant improvement. That's why the cosmetic dermatological mountain is such a slippery slope for consumers to navigate — there is no clear path in sight. When I asked celebrity dermatologist Dr. Patricia Wexler about going in one direction versus another, she told me, "There are many ways to get downtown." (She admits that she's not the first doctor to use that expression!) If a doctor suggests the same laser as the answer to a variety of your problems, be wary. It may be the only laser in his or her office. "The worst thing you can do is to use inappropriate technology," warns Dr. Neil Sadick, whose Sadick Dermatology Center in New York is a showcase for state-of-the-art treatment. "When someone turns their laser on you for the wrong reason, that can lead to poor results," he says. Before undergoing any treatment, he suggests that you do your homework, going so far as

to check your doctor's credentials with respected groups such as the American Society of Laser Medicine Surgery (aslms.org) and the American Academy of Cosmetic Surgery (cosmeticsurgery .org). You can't be too careful; this is your face.

Because next-generation technologies are always in development, you're bound to encounter new options once you're in the doctor's office. "Every month there's something new," confirms my friend and dermatologist Dr. Gervaise Gerstner. Unless you have a subscription to the *Journal of the American Academy of Dermatology,* it's almost impossible to keep up on all this. But ultimately it's your call whether you allow something to be injected into your face. Don't hesitate to ask your doctor for more information so that you can do some research before you commit. I know that it's hard to say no once you're sitting in the office, but you have to have the guts to do just that if your doctor is suggesting something that makes you nervous. I'm reminded of the time I once went to interview a plastic surgeon, who said, "I have half a syringe of Botox left over from another patient. Want some? It's free!" I know he was trying to be nice, but I wasn't prepared to have Botox yet — free or otherwise — so I said, "No, thanks." Remember, you can always exercise your option of getting up and walking out.

Your "Refreshing" Menu

By the time you read this, there will most likely be several new Next Big Things, but it still pays to familiarize yourself with some of those that have become standard dermatological practice.

Lasers: Lasers are machines that use light or heat to improve the skin. Different lasers serve different purposes, but most doctors now use only those that fall into the "non-ablative" category. Ablative lasers, such as CO_2 and erbium: YAG lasers, are considered old-fashioned. They literally take off layers of skin, leaving you looking like a burn victim for weeks or months. They can also leave you looking glisteningly gooey and healing patchily (hypopigmentation). The newer, non-ablative versions, such as the Fraxel Skin Resurfacing laser, can be used to eliminate age spots, scars, and uneven texture with a few days of recovery.

Peels: Better exfoliation through chemistry. One of the quickest, easiest, and least painful things you can have done at the dermatologist's is a light chemical peel (glycolic, TCA, for example). "If someone isn't exactly sure of what they want to do, but they know they want something, they book a light peel," says Dr. Gerstner. A popular treatment is a series of six glycolic acid peels (about one a month) that increase in strength (from a 20 percent to a 70 percent solution). The results will be subtle, but getting peels done on a regular basis will help speed cell turnover, so that skin tone and texture improve, and fine lines and dark spots may get less noticeable. There are medium and deep chemical peels, too, but they can't be considered quick, easy, and painless.

Microdermabrasion: Whereas peels use a chemical (such as glycolic acid) to get skin to shed its dead cells, microdermabrasion is exfoliation by machine, which mechanically scrubs skin off using very fine crystals. Again, a series of treatments is usually recommended to improve skin tone, texture, dark spots, scarring, and fine lines.

LED (Light Emitting Diode) Photomodulation: From brands such as Gentle Waves, an easy "lunchtime" treatment that involves sitting in front of a panel of intense bright lights (a narrow band of light-emitting diodes) that pulsate across your face for forty-five seconds, producing firmer, plumper, more elastic skin. It's very futuristic and doesn't hurt a bit — except that it can set you back $1,500 for eight 45-second treatments.

Injectables: Good old-fashioned Botox is the gold standard for removing fine lines, since the injections effectively freeze the muscles that cause you to squint or furrow. The treatment is quick and not terribly painful, and the results are visible almost immediately (it can take up to two weeks for the full "freeze" to take place). Results typically last only about three to six months, but some doctors claim that if you have regular Botox injections, the results are cumulative, allowing you to go longer between injections until you don't need them anymore.

There is an arsenal of fillers available to plump up your wrinkles and fill your lines. Plus, new (and hopefully improved) injectables are awaiting approval from the FDA. Of course, the drug companies are marketing these directly to consumers, and you may be tempted to ask for one by name. It's good to know what's out there, but your doctor will have an opinion regarding which one is best for you based on his or her experience with it, where it's going, how long it will last, and how much it costs.

Fat: Using your own fat to fill in wrinkles sounds like a great idea: take it from where you don't need it, and put it where you do! Doctors disagree about how long fat lasts, and it has to be injected quite deep with a big needle in order to last at all.

Human collagen: Products such as CosmoDerm (for fine lines) and CosmoPlast (a thicker formula for deeper lines) are made from human collagen. Advantage: It doesn't require a test for allergies.

Bovine collagen: Zyderm and Zyplast are made from cow collagen. ArteFill is a perma-nent filler that is a mixture of bovine collagen with lidocaine and polymethylmethacrylate (PMMA). Disadvantage: It requires a test for allergies. That it can last up to nine years can be an advantage and disadvantage. (See the silicone entry.)

Hyaluronic acid: Restylane, Juvaderm, Captique, and Hylaform are made from this natural sugar. Perlane, the latest filler in this group to receive FDA approval, is a hyaluronic acid compound similar to Restylane, and both are touted to last for up to a year.

Silicone: Silikon 1000 is a more permanent filler that can last for three years or longer. Advan-tage: You don't have to get it redone every few months. Disad-vantage: If anything goes wrong, you're stuck with it. "Permanent fillers equal permanent complica-tions," says Dr. Gerstner, who won't use permanent fillers for that reason.

Synthetic poly-L-lactic acid: Sculptra is a long-lasting filler (up to two years) to pump up aging faces. Injections take several sessions and may leave bumps.

RESET THE CLOCK AT THE DERM
"There are things that can be done to slow down the biological clock," says Dr. Sadick. "We can tighten your skin without surgery. We have light surfaces that stimulate collagen on a long-term basis. We can turn over your skin cells." Although it's easy to get excited about the possibilities, it's best not to attempt to do everything at once, or you run the risk of looking like a Woman Who Has Had Too Much Work Done. So before you see your doctor, decide what is really bothering you. Dr. Wexler's first question to every new patient is, "What's your skin concern?" Is it the furrow in your forehead that makes you look as if you're always angry? The sagging skin under your chin that keeps you in compensatory necklines? The brown splotches and ruddiness on your face? Have a few small tweaks at a time, so that all anyone notices is that you seem to look less tired, more relaxed, refreshed, and wonderfully Y&H! When looking for a skin guru, Dr. Gerstner advises, "Find a doctor who will go slowly. If they don't go slowly, run!"

THERE'S HOMEWORK TO DO
Even Dr. Sadick, who helps develop over-the-counter skin care products for Dior, confirms that there are limits to the kind of dramatic results you can get with an over-the-counter cream or serum. "Are you talking about erasing deep wrinkles? Absolutely not," he says. "Are you talking about smoothing fine wrinkles and slowing down the wrinkling process? Absolutely yes. Hydrating the skin, stimulating new collagen, and decreasing redness are realistic goals." Women spend an es-timated $470 million a year on antiaging products, but simply spending more isn't necessarily going to buy you any better ammunition for your battle against wrinkles. According to *Consumer Re-ports' Shop Smart* magazine, which tested nine wrinkle creams at various price points, some of

the most effective (Olay) were drugstore brands, while some of the least effective (La Prairie) cost hundreds of dollars.

The role of at-home products is maintenance. Whether or not you choose to see a dermatologist, getting religion about daily skin care is essential. "You need to have a program," advises Dr. Sadick, who thinks that you can keep it simple. "If you want to have healthy skin, protect it with a high-dose antioxidant and a sunblock every morning. At night, turn over your skin. I truly believe you can turn back the clock at least a decade on wrinkles at night." Here's a five-step program.

1. Cleanse: Keeping your skin clean — free of dirt, bacteria, and makeup — will go a long way toward keeping it looking fresh. Choose a gentle cleanser that won't strip your skin (your face shouldn't feel tight after you wash it). I like Patricia Wexler M.D. Universal Anti-Aging Cleanser. In fact, I love her entire skin care line. My other Brilliant Buys include Clarins Cleansing Milk with Alpine Herbs, because it's so soft and creamy it almost makes you want

If You Have . . .

✔**Crow's-feet**
You could try: Botox. It will relax the lines, and if they aren't too deep, this may be enough to make them nearly disappear. Wait a couple of weeks after a Botox injection, and if the lines still bother you, your doctor can use an injectable filler, such as CosmoDerm, to plump them up.

✔**Frown lines**
You could try: Botox. The protocol is pretty much the same as for crow's-feet. You need to relax the muscles to keep you from furrowing, then fill any remaining deeper lines with one of the fillers.

✔**Smile lines**
You could try: A collagen filler such as CosmoDerm or Zyderm. To plump up these lines on the sides of your mouth (nasolabial folds), doctors often employ a layering technique. This adds volume and gives long-lasting results.

✔**Neck jowls**
You could try: Botox plus Thermage (a noninvasive treatment that uses radio frequencies), which purportedly helps tighten skin by inducing collagen contraction and promoting new collagen growth. Thermage is expensive ($1,000 to $5,000), and although it promises that you'll "get back the real you," there's no guarantee that either it or Botox will tame a true turkey neck.

✔**Lip lines**
You could try: A Fraxel laser or a filler such as CosmoDerm. The non-ablative laser can help erase lines as it resurfaces your skin. The filler can help plump them up so they aren't so noticeable. (See chapter 9 for more details.)

✔**Dark spots or uneven skin tone**
(that can't be covered by foundation)
You could try: Microdermabrasion or chemical peels. Mild cases might see improvement as these relatively easy treatments remove a few layers of skin. More serious spots will require laser resurfacing.

✔**Broken capillaries**
You could try: A laser. These spidery little clusters that often show up around the nose and scream OL can be zapped away quickly with a laser.

Buyer Beware: Who Is Wielding the Syringe?

The biggest controversy in the world of cosmetic procedures is the debate over who should be allowed to wield the syringe. A growing number of doctors who are not dermatologists or plastic surgeons are cashing in on this lucrative field by offering Botox, fillers, and laser treatments to their patients. Although many of the gynecologists, family practitioners, urologists, dentists, and other medical professionals who take continuing education seminars see nothing wrong with venturing into aesthetic procedures, some critics warn that doctors practicing outside their expertise is inherently risky. It's best to put your face in the hands of a doctor with years of experience and training in dermatology or plastic surgery.

The other area of debate is the "medi-spa," which may be a euphemism for the old-fashioned beauty parlor down the street or a storefront clinic sometimes found even in shopping malls. The danger is that these medi-spas often have aestheticians administer injections and do laser treatments with (or without) a doctor on the premises. The term "doctor on premises" gives a false sense of security, because it doesn't mean all that much if the doctor isn't the one with the syringe. Although all these treatments may seem virtually harmless, stories of procedures gone wrong abound. So go to these places for a facial or a massage, but see a dermatologist or plastic surgeon for anything more involved.

to wash your face before you hit the pillow, and Philosophy Purity Made Simple, which removes eye makeup at the same time. Cetaphil Gentle Skin Cleanser is always a winner.

2. Exfoliate: As we get older, our skin cells don't turn over as rapidly as they once did, resulting in a rough, uneven, or blotchy texture. To speed up cell turnover and help reveal fresher-looking skin, you need to give those cells a nudge. One of the first (and still best) at-home microdermabrasion kits is the L'Oréal Paris Advanced RevitaLift Micro-Dermabrasion Kit, which you can use a few times a week. If you prefer not to scrub, you can use Patricia Wexler M.D. Dermatology Exfoliating Glyco Peel System daily, unless your skin is super-sensitive. For a heated masklike treat, I like Olay Regenerist Thermal Skin Polisher. This unique product is a scrub with glycolic acid that warms up on your face and is gentle enough to use daily.

3. Restore: A dizzying number of antioxidants seem to take turns on the hot list, each promising to reverse the damage already done and to perform other skin-saving miracles.

Every morning, slap on a serum, a rich cocktail delivering potent doses of skin-fixing vitamins. You want an antioxidant-rich product, such as Elizabeth Arden Prevage Anti-Aging Treatment. Studies have shown that antioxidants can help boost skin's defenses against damaging free radicals. I am crazy about Patricia Wexler M.D. Dermatology MMPi Skin Regenerating Serum, which looks like pink Vaseline and feels like cashmere on your cheeks.

At night, nothing has been proven to restore your skin like prescription Retin-A, aka Renova. It has withstood the test of time (as well as clinical testing) and consistently works to improve skin tone and texture and even help build collagen. You can get drugstore products that contain retinol, but they aren't as potent as the prescription version. You can't use Retin-A every night (every other

(PLEASE DON'T . . .) Underestimate the effects of your lifestyle on your skin. Dr. Gerstner tells all her patients that the most important things they can do for their skin are to wear sunscreen, not to smoke, to maintain a healthy body weight, and not to yo-yo diet. "A full, round face is youthful. Go back to your high school yearbook and look how full your cheeks were," she says. "A thin, gaunt face will make you look old."

night is suggested), so switch off with a cream that will really make a difference in the morning. My favorites include Clinique Turnaround Concentrate Visible Skin Renewer, Elizabeth Arden Prevage Anti-Aging Treatment, Guerlain Orchidée Impériale Cream, and Patricia Wexler M.D. Dermatology Intensive Night Reversal and Repair Cream.

4. Moisturize: When skin is dry, even fine lines start to look like wrinkles etched deep into the skin — a very OL look for sure. By adding moisture to your skin, you can temporarily plump it up, making it look dewier and more youthful. Moisturizers that cost a mint, such as celebrity favorite Crème de la Mer, Shiseido Future Solution, and Guerlain Orchidée Impériale Cream, are wonderfully luxurious, but you can also get good results from less pricey products. Whenever someone complains to me about the high price of skin care, I tell them to buy Olay Definity Deep Penetrating Foaming Moisturizer. I love its mousse-like texture. If you don't want to slap on yet another product, make sure your daily moisturizer multitasks as a sunscreen. At the drugstore, Dr. Gerstner recommends Olay Complete Defense SPF 30 Daily UV Moisturizer. If you're near a Bath & Body Works, check out Patricia Wexler M.D. Dermatology Universal Anti-Aging Moisturizer or Skin Brightening Daily Moisturizer, both SPF 30.

5. Protect: If your moisturizer doesn't include a sunscreen, add one more product to your routine. Sunscreen (at least SPF 15 every day) is essential not only for preventing skin cancer but also for defending against the UV damage that leads to signs of aging. If you're going on vacation and plan to play a lot of tennis, golf, or water sports, splurge on La Roche-Posay Anthelios SX Daily Moisturizing Cream with Mexoryl SX SPF 15 (it goes up to SPF 60). What is Mexoryl? It provides peak efficacy, blocking short UVA rays as well as UVB rays. And if you decide to have a peel, microdermabrasion, or laser resurfacing to get rid of brown spots, stay out of the sun or slather on even more sunscreen. Without protection, those dark patches you paid good money to eradicate are going to come right back. "Your skin is smart, and it remembers them," says Dr. Gerstner. "After fifteen minutes in the sun without protection, those spots will reappear."

HIGH, MEDIUM, AND LOW MAINTENANCE . . . ANTIAGING TREATMENTS

Okay, science class is almost dismissed, but by now you have a pretty good idea of what you can do to fight back against wrinkles and telltale OL signs. Here's a quick recap of how these treatments rank in terms of maintenance.

HIGH: You know you're high maintenance if your primary physician is your derm. Your quarterly visits include laser, LED, and a combo platter of fillers and freezers.

MEDIUM: You seek out newer, longer-lasting injectables so you'll end up spending less time and money at the doctor. Also, doing just one thing — Botox only on your frown lines, for example — qualifies as medium maintenance. And while you're at the derm, sign on for a series of glycolic acid peels. Your skin will look decidedly fresher for a minimal investment.

LOW: Buy new products that deliver the best results possible. How about a retinol regimen, plus skin treats from the highly regarded Olay Regenerist or Definity line? Remember that the best things you can do for your skin fall under low mainte-nance: use sunscreen, don't smoke, and don't get too thin in the face!

LAST BUT NOT LEAST: UNDER YOUR EYES

You can tell the difference between a thirty-year-old and a fifty-year-old by looking at the skin under their eyes. The thirty-year-old may still be dewy and fresh; the fifty-year-old is likely to have dark circles and per-manent puffiness. If you started late on eye cream, or if under-eye aging just runs in your family, you might have to step up your plan of action. To lighten up the discoloration, ask your dermatologist about Restylane. Those hollow, dark circles, often resulting in shadows, may disappear when plumped up. To remove those pads of fat which give you puffiness, see a plastic surgeon about a lower lid blepharoplas-ty (see chapter 6, page 58). Neither choice is fast and easy, but hey, at least you have options.

B R I L L I A N T   B U Y S

CLEANSERS
Cetaphil Gentle Skin Cleanser, $10.50; drugstores and mass retailers
Clarins Cleansing Milk with Alpine Herbs, $27; clarins.com
Kiehl's Ultra Moisturizing Cleansing Cream, $20.50; kiehls.com
Olay Regenerist Daily Regenerating Cleanser, $7.99; drugstores and mass retailers
Patricia Wexler M.D. Dermatology Universal Anti-Aging Cleanser, $18; Bath & Body Works, 800-756-5005 or bathandbodyworks.com
philosophy Purity Made Simple (8 oz.), $20; Sephora, 877-737-4672 or sephora.com; philosophy.com

EXFOLIATORS
L'Oréal Paris Advanced RevitaLift Micro-Dermabrasion Kit, $24.99; drugstores and mass retailers
Olay Regenerist Microdermabrasion & Peel Kit, $25; drugstores and mass retailers
Olay Regenerist Thermal Skin Pol-isher, $13.99; drugstores and mass retailers
Patricia Wexler M.D. Dermatology Exfoliating Glyco Peel System, $65; Bath & Body Works, 800-756-5005 or bathandbodyworks.com

RESTORING TREATMENTS
Dermalogica Multivitamin Power Concentrate, $52; dermalogica.com
Elizabeth Arden Prevage Anti-Aging Treatment, $150; elizabetharden.com
Estée Lauder Idealist Pore Minimiz-ing Skin Refinisher, $46.50; Saks, 877-551-7257; esteelauder.com
Garnier Nutritioniste Ultra-Lift Serum, $14.99; drugstores and mass retailers
Kiehl's Powerful-Strength Line-Reducing Concentrate, $55; kiehls.com
Patricia Wexler M.D. Dermatology MMPi Skin Regenerating Serum, $55; Bath & Body Works, 800-756-5005 or bathandbodyworks.com
Good Skin Smooth-365 Intensive Clarity + Smoothing Peptite Serum, $42.50; Kohls, kohls.com
Tracie Martyn Firming Serum, $185; traciemartyn.com

EYE CREAMS

Olay Regenerist Eye Derma-Pod Anti-Aging Triple Response System, $27.99; drugstores and mass retailers

Prescriptives Anti-Age Advanced Protection Lotion SPF 25, $60; prescriptives.com

MOISTURIZERS

Crème de La Mer (1oz.), $110; lamer.com

Estée Lauder Hydra Complete Multi-Level Moisture Creme for Dry Skin, $40; Saks, 877-551-7257; esteelauder.com

Guerlain Orchidée Impériale Cream, $360; Neiman Marcus, 888-888-4757; Saks, saks.com

Guerlain Orchidée Impériale Fluid, $250; Neiman Marcus, 888-888-4757; Saks, saks.com

La Mer The Moisturizing Lotion (1.7 oz.), $165; lamer.com

Olay Complete Defense SPF 30 Daily UV Moisturizer, $13.99; drugstores and mass retailers

Olay Definity Deep Penetrating Foaming Moisturizer, $28.99; drugstores and mass retailers

Patricia Wexler M.D. Dermatology Skin Brightening Daily Moisturizer, $39.50; Bath & Body Works, 800-756-5005 or bathandbodyworks.com

Patricia Wexler M.D. Dermatology Universal Anti-Aging Moisturizer SPF 30+, $39.50; Bath & Body Works, 800-756-5005 or bathandbodyworks.com

Shiseido Bio-Performance Advanced Super Revitalizer Cream (1.7 oz.), $70; Macy's, 800-289-6229 or macys.com

Shiseido Future Solution Total Revitalizing Cream (1.8 oz.), $225; Macy's, 800-289-6229 or macys.com

DAYTIME WRINKLE SMOOTHER

Clarins Instant Smooth Perfecting Touch, $27; clarins.com

Patricia Wexler M.D. Dermatology Advanced Fastscription No-Injection Wrinkle Smoother, $29.50; Bath & Body Works, 800-756-5005 or bathandbodyworks.com

NIGHTTIME WRINKLE ERASERS

Renova, by prescription only

Clinique Turnaround Concentrate Visible Skin Renewer, $36.50; Bloomingdale's, 800-555-7467; clinique.com

Patricia Wexler M.D. Dermatology Intensive Night Reversal & Repair Cream, $42.50; Bath & Body Works, 800-756-5005 or bathandbodyworks.com

MASK

Estée Lauder Idealist Micro-D Deep Thermal Refinisher, $46; Saks, 877-551-7257; esteelauder.com

SUNSCREEN

La Roche-Posay Anthelios SX Daily Moisturizing Cream with Mexoryl SX SPF 15, $29; anthelios.com or CVS

9

PUT ON PINK

LIPSTICK

NOTHING AGES YOU LIKE . . .
DARK LIPSTICK . . . LIPSTICK BLEEDING INTO FINE LINES . . . CRACKED LIPS . . . THIN LIPS . . . OBVIOUS LIP LINER . . . OVERLY MATTE LIPSTICK . . . OBVIOUSLY FAKE PLUMPED LIPS

If you need proof that pink is the only lipstick color worth wearing, just think of Angelina Jolie. She is, after all, the woman whose lips are most requested in cosmetic surgeons' offices, whose career was launched in part on the power of her pout, who is believed by both men and women to be among the sexiest creatures on earth, who could get away with wearing any color lipstick. So what does she paint on her lips? Most of the time, whether she's walking on the red carpet or just being a mom, Angelina wears a light, glossy pink.

Why succumb to the power of pink? Because — and this is true for women of all skin tones — the right pink lightens up the mouth with a shimmery luminosity that helps compensate for the loss of glow in our complexions. The rare times Angelina is photographed in another color, it's usually for a movie in which she is supposed to look older.

Isn't a bright red lip more dramatic and attention grabbing? Yes, but who wants to draw all that attention to her lips? Iconic Paloma Picasso pulls off fiery red with pizzazz, but don't kid yourself — it's tough to wear! Darker lip colors emphasize the dark circles under eyes. And the darker the color, the thinner your lips will look. You can apply the same principle of dark and light from fashion: darker minimizes; lighter emphasizes. If you're feeling heavy, are you going to slip on black or white pants? You're going to choose black, because black makes your butt look smaller. By contrast, you want your lips to be fat, so choose the white pants equivalent: pink helps plump them up!

There's a practical reason to make the switch to pink lipstick: lip lines. I hate lip lines, those tiny (well, maybe not so tiny), vertical crevices that show up one day on your lips and keep getting deeper. I don't even want to think about how much money I've spent trying to get rid of them. And when those telltale lines meet up with dark lipstick, the result isn't pretty. If you know what I'm talking about, you have experienced "settling," when dark lipstick finds its way into those crevices, and they become even more obvious. And what about when dark lipstick "bleeds" up over your lip? I can live with it when it happens with a glossy pink but not with a deep burgundy.

So now what? Purge your lipstick collection of all those evil dark shades — and the matching lip liners they came with. (Lipsticks only have a shelf life of four years anyway.) If you're having second thoughts about tossing, here is makeup artist Nick Barose to convince you otherwise.

■ "**Mauve** makes you look older and sad."

■ "**Nudes** can make you look like a washed-out zombie."

■ "**Orange** veers into the clownish."

■ "**Purples** make you look like you're suffering from hypothermia."

Okay?

YOUR POWER POUT: WHICH SHADE OF PINK?

If the pink is too dark, it will blend into your lip color. If it's too light, it will wash you out. As you try the buffet of pinks, you'll see that a pink one or two shades lighter than your natural lip color shines just the right spotlight.

This is a time you may want to seek professional help. Park yourself down in a chair at your favorite makeup counter and let a pro suggest the best pinks for you. Then you can edit the choices down to The One. I know that most women loathe department store makeup counters, because the sales associates who work on commission are always pushing, pushing, pushing. They're intimidating and make you feel guilty about what you're not willing to spend. You walk away with a charge on your credit card just because you feel as if you have to save face. Is it any wonder that Sephora is such a success? (What a concept: a retailer that encourages you to walk around and try products by providing all the little amenities — applicators, makeup remover, cotton balls, tissues, and mirrors!)

Back to the department store: your challenge (should you choose to buy your pink lipstick there) is to find one fabulous sales associate whom you can bond with (it's like finding a partner, you only need one!). Ask for the best makeup artist at the counter and start there. The bonus of doing this research while you're out shopping is that the next time you have a special event to go to, where you want to get a little more dolled up, you'll have his or her card so you can call and make an appointment. The fact that you've already road tested this person will reduce the margin of error (and increase your confidence), and you won't have to worry about how you're going to look fabulous. The makeup counter is a medium-maintenance way to get a high-maintenance look. (Hiring a makeup artist to come to your house can run $200 or more.) If, after a couple of visits, you absolutely love how you look, ask if you can get a private makeup lesson. (You may want to do this in the privacy of your home rather than in the middle of the busy cosmetic department.)

As mentioned earlier, at mass retailers such as Target or your local Rite-Aid, you may be able to return a shade if you take it home and discover it's not right. (Since all the chains have different policies, ask customer service before you buy.) If you can't decide between two colors, take both. Who can't use two tubes of pink lipstick?

In your quest for the perfect pink, texture counts. Look for lipsticks that are creamy. Long-wearing formulas have improved over the years, but some may still be too drying, which will only accentuate and exacerbate lip lines. Stay away from lip stains. Although they're sheer and pretty, they're formulated to stain (that is, last a long time) and can gather in the creases. They won't smooth over your lips, and they won't add enough shine. And don't go matte or opaque either. Susan Sterling, Chanel's international makeup artist, cautions that because matte lipsticks have no light-reflecting shine, they accentuate the lines around your mouth. Your best bet, according to both Susan and Nick Barose, is a lipstick that's velvety with a hint of sheen. Nick opines, "Opaque lipstick is about as youthful as opaque nude panty hose!"

LIP SERVICE: FOUR STEPS TO THE PERFECT POUT

Full disclosure: I don't take twenty minutes to create the perfectly precise lip like makeup artists do — and like they tell you to do. More often than not, I don't even have time to put lipstick on before I leave the house. So I take it with me to do en route, either in the back of a cab or while my husband is driving us to a movie or party. Here's my down-and-dirty, fast way to fabulous lips.

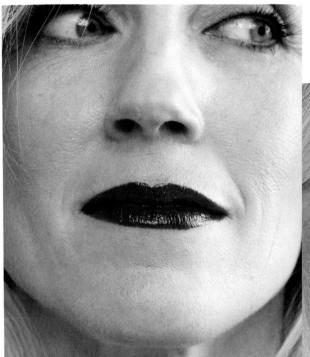

TOO OLD: dark lips look so OL

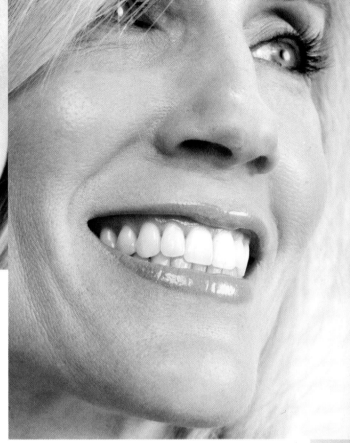

JUST RIGHT: a quick switch to shimmery pink is Y&H

1. Prep the lips: Exfoliate and moisturize. This is the first thing to do when applying makeup. There's no sense in laying all that gorgeous color over a cracked, dry, peeling surface. (You wouldn't do that to a wall!) For one thing, it looks bad. For another, the lipstick won't adhere well. To remove all those flaky bits, gently rub a specially formulated lip exfoliator over your lips. Some lip exfoliators are moisturizers as well, but if yours is not, coat your lips with lip balm so they'll be plump and ready to hold the color. This is the first step in your makeup routine, because you want the moisturizer to settle in while you do the rest of your face. When you get to your lips, they'll be primed and ready.

2. Conceal the evidence: Dot concealer along the edge of your upper lip (or wherever you have lip lines). This will fill in the lines and prevent lipstick from feathering into them. Concealer provides a bit of a barrier to keep your lipstick from bailing on you.

3. Shape it up: I hope you're not one of those women who outline their lips in a dark color, then fill in with lipstick that's lighter than the lip liner. Could anything be more OL? If you're using a lip liner to give the illusion of a fuller lip, no one should

know. So why would you wear a lip liner that's darker than your lip color? I don't know how this trend started, but even Jerry Seinfeld commented on it in his documentary *Comedian:* "There are some trends I'm looking forward to coming to an end. Ladies, the outline around the lips is over. I wish I could just say to all the women on behalf of the men of Planet Earth — *We see your lips!*" Okay, Jerry, you said it!

The truth is, the older you get, the more you

Nick Barose is going to let you in on a little trick he learned from Kim Cattrall. The secret is to limit your liner just to where you need it.

need lip liner. It helps define your lips, keeps them from disappearing, and can make them appear fuller and shapelier. (Angelina, here we come.)

Your lip liner should be either the exact color of your lips or one or two shades lighter so you'll never get caught with a dark line around your lips. Our lips often lose pigmentation over the years, so when you lighten up your lipstick, lighten up your lip liner, too. What I once considered my neutrals — Chanel Le Crayon Lèvres Precision Lip Definer in Nude and MAC Lip Pencil in Spice — are now too dark, and I've had to switch to Chanel Lip Definer in Tawny and MAC Cremestick Liner in Cream O' Spice. Line your lips "the newer way" (at right), and after you've shaped them, fill in both lips, upper and lower, with the liner, just as if you were coloring in a cartoon. This will help your lipstick adhere better and last longer. And if it still bails on you, at least you're covered in liner.

4. Add color: Here you have two choices — lipstick or gloss. Lipstick lasts longer than gloss, but if applied with a brush, it takes longer to put on. The pros of gloss? It catches the light, making your lips look plumper and therefore younger. (I love Chanel Lèvres Scintillantes Glossimer in Rose Sand. It's a classic, shimmery baby pink.) The cons? Gloss requires frequent reapplications. Your call. If you're going the lipstick route, you can add one dot of gloss afterward, in the center of your bottom lip, to further the illusion of plumpness. Done: your perfect pink pout!

The Newer Way to . . .
Line Your Lips
Chances are you have a perfectly fine bottom lip; most women do. It's the upper lip that's the prob-

lem. The top lip is the one that thins most notice-ably in both width and plumpness (loss of colla-gen). To get the lushest lips possible, Nick Barose is going to let you in on a little trick he learned from Kim Cattrall. The secret is to limit your liner just to where you need it. The result? So much more Y&H. (Thanks, Kim!)

■ **If your top lip is still full** and well shaped, you can concentrate on the bow of the lip, giving it a little definition by following its natural line.

■ **If the top lip has thinned out,** give it the illu-sion of volume by starting in the middle of one side and arching up toward the bow about a centime-ter or so above your actual lip line. When you get to the bow, cheat nature a little and draw more pronounced peaks, then arch back down to the middle of the other side.

■ **If your bottom lip gets lost underneath** your top lip, just line the bottom lip.

■ **If your entire lip needs plumping,** try not to make one continuous line circling your entire mouth — too obvious. Draw broken lines instead.

TOO DARK: Sharon Stone in matte red . . .

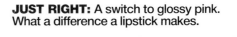

JUST RIGHT: A switch to glossy pink. What a difference a lipstick makes.

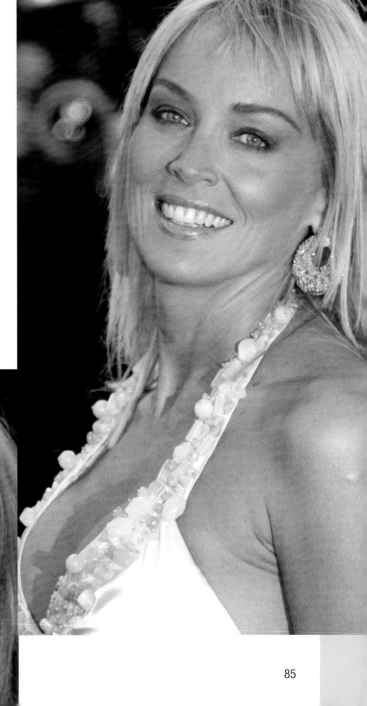

85

💲 Is It Worth It?

💲 **Lip Plumpers.** Almost every beauty line now has a $20 to $50 lip enhancer promising fuller lips. Here's the deal: The newer ones that give you a slight tingling are better than the older ones that require you to massage a cream or serum into your lips for at least a minute. The very act of rubbing your lips irritates them and causes them to inflate a bit. With the best plumpers, you may see your lips plump up temporarily. The key word being "temporarily," which may mean for an hour or two. Dr. Gervaise Gerstner advises, "Don't waste a penny. They're like cellulite reducers — totally temporary." As for getting collagen injections in your lips (as opposed to the tiny lines above them), you run the risk of having your lips look like a pucker fish, as immortalized by Goldie Hawn in *The First Wives Club.* You're much better off plumping your lip line with liner and lipstick.

HIGH, MEDIUM, AND LOW MAINTENANCE . . . FILLING IN LIP LINES

Vertical cracks that take up residence above the upper lip are a problem I know well. I also know that over-the-counter beauty balms — even $250 ones — don't fill in deep lines. Whether they are caused by smoking or facial expressions or are just a hereditary gift from your parents, these lines scream OL. (I've never smoked, so I'm convinced my lines came from years of pursing my lips to drink Diet Coke out of the can three times a day.) I'm not convinced that the perfect solution is out there yet, but if you mind the gaps, here's what you can do until it comes along.

HIGH: The Fraxel laser is a non-ablative tool that targets cells under the skin to regenerate collagen production. It is designed to work in six sessions, at a cost of $1,500 per session. It produces results but leaves you red-faced and swollen. Recovery after each session can take up to a week. It is not a permanent solution, lasting roughly only six months (for $9,000, thank you). I don't recommend the heavy artillery of the CO_2 laser, but it does work. Used for complete resurfacing, it strips skin to its bottom layer. It's a real ordeal, can cause hypopigmentation, and requires significant downtime. My sister walked around looking like a burn victim for four months after her CO_2 treatment. Yes, her lip lines are gone, but was it worth it? Not to me.

MEDIUM: CosmoDerm or CosmoPlast are collagen fillers that are injected by a dermatologist into the lines to plump them up. Upside: They tend to work well. Downside: They last only two to six months. "We use our lips all the time," explains Dr. Gerstner. "They're just not going to hold filler for a long time." She says people often beg her to use silicone because it is considered permanent, but she and many other doctors refuse to go there. As she said earlier, "Permanent fillers equal permanent complications." The average price of one syringe of CosmoDerm or CosmoPlast is $400.

LOW: Retinol creams made from retinoic acid work at a cellular level, spurring cells to create more collagen and therefore plump up the skin and decrease the appearance of lines. The upside is that they are the only topical treatment (so far) that can soften lines and make them appear less visible. (That's not to say your lines will disappear.) The downside is that these products take a while to produce results. See your dermatologist for prescription creams with Retin-A such as Renova, which have the strongest percentage of retinol. Or look for over-the-counter options at the drugstore or a mass retailer.

Everywhere you want hair, it's thinning. Everywhere you don't want hair, it's growing.

GOOD-BYE TO LIP (AND CHIN) HAIR

On her 2006 HBO special, Roseanne Barr joked about the joys of aging: "Everywhere you want to be wet, you're dry. Everywhere you want to be dry, you're wet." To that I would add: "Everywhere you want hair, it's thinning. Everywhere you don't want hair, it's growing." During menopause, when hormone levels are in flux, many women notice more hair than usual on the upper lip and chin. Nothing looks more OL than a mustache and chin hairs, so they must be removed immediately — but how?

The old-fashioned way is with wax. I was indoctrinated into the world of wax in grade school when sitting in the kitchen of my best friend, Gayle. Her mother urged us to eat Popsicles so that she could use the wooden sticks afterward to apply the pea green wax boiling on the burner to her upper lip. Yum-o! In high school, my mother, sister, and I had a double boiler dedicated to the hot yellow wax that the three of us used. Talk about a bonding experience! In the years since, I've jumped from low to high maintenance when it comes to facial hair removal. TMI (too much information), for sure, so let's just talk about your options for coming clean.

HIGH, MEDIUM, AND LOW MAINTENANCE . . . ZAPPING FACIAL HAIR

HIGH: Laser hair reduction, if you're a good candidate, is the only way to go. It zaps hundreds of hairs in a single session, and once gone, they're not coming back — or at least they're not coming back very fast. In the first session, the laser weakens the hair follicle by targeting it with heat. After a full course of treatment (usually five to seven sessions), the follicle becomes permanently disabled and unable to grow hair. Although lasers are better than virtually anything else out there, they're not perfect. Since they can only get rid of hair that exists at the time of treatment, any hair that is dormant during your session may show up later. (This is why the FDA-approved term is "laser hair reduction," not removal.) Additionally, if you experience a hormone shift after you have been through all the sessions, hairs may sprout where they never existed before. Terri Levin, an R.N. and nurse-practitioner on Long Island who works extensively with lasers, explains that "you're not stopping the underlying cause; you're just stopping the hairs that are there today." Many women may need another session or two after the initial series for upkeep. If only a few hairs spring up later, it may be more practical for you to tweeze or shave them away (see low maintenance).

Before you commit, make sure that you're an appropriate candidate for the laser that will be used. Most lasers work by seeking out contrast between skin color and hair color. So if you have light skin and dark facial hair (or whatever kind of hair you want removed), you're in luck. If, however, you have light skin and light hair, this process is not going to work, and you'll have to resort to the lower-maintenance options. Similarly, if you have extremely dark skin and dark hair, it might be a no go. This is not to say that all African American women should forget about laser hair removal. The FDA has approved many lasers for use on dark skin, but women with skin as dark as their hair are likely to be wasting their money. Ditto for women with light skin and fair hair. In these cases, the laser cannot "see" the hair.

The pain factor can be minimized by applying a numbing cream such as Emla to the area for about an hour prior to the treatment. You can and should get a prescription for this before your first appointment so that you can apply it before you arrive at the office and not waste time waiting for it to kick in.

Lasers are not risk-free. If used incorrectly, they can burn you, which is why it's so unfortunate that the field is virtually unregulated. Anyone can set up shop, and as the technique has gained in popularity — and gotten more profitable — people without proper training have done just that. So before you let anyone approach your face with such a powerful high-tech weapon, do your research. Ideally, you should find someone trained in the medical field, either as a doctor, nurse practitioner, or a nurse. The medical pro should ask if you are taking any medications (this can be a factor in how your skin reacts to the laser), and you should ask him or her how many times he or she has done the procedure. You want someone who's done it hundreds of times. Inquire about his or her experience with your particular skin type and color and whether the laser is FDA approved. This is impor-

tant for all women, but especially for women of color, because hypopigmentation is a danger.

Charges are commonly assessed per area. For example, the chin, lip, and brow are considered separate areas. On average, each area costs $200 per session, and five to seven sessions are needed.

MEDIUM: Get waxed by a pro. You leave the cleanup to someone else, and you can be sure she won't flinch at the idea of violently ripping hair from your face (or other body parts). Just because it's low-tech, however, doesn't mean it can't burn. If you're using Retin-A, are taking certain medications, or have recently had a laser procedure or peel, your skin is going to be too sensitive and raw for waxing. The cost for both the upper lip and the chin is about $7 to $20 each.

Another medium-maintenance option is electrolysis, although it's so old-school that electrolysis technicians are now renting laser equipment. Electrolysis eliminates hairs one by one, as opposed to a number of hairs at once, so it is incredibly labor-intensive and time-consuming, requiring far more sessions. If you just have a few stubborn hairs to get rid of permanently, it's worth considering. The cost starts around $25 per area per session.

LOW: Tweezing, home waxing, depilatories, and shaving are all low-cost alternatives. A lot of women bristle at the mere mention of shaving because it's such a guy thing, but it is an easy, effective option, and compared to waxing and depilatories, it's mess-free. Contrary to popular belief, it will not cause hair to grow in any faster, but it will create stubble, which can feel coarse. All of these options cost less than $20 at the drugstore.

LIP CONDITIONER
C.O. Bigelow Mentha Lip Shine, $7.50; Bath & Body Works, 800-756-5005 or bathandbodyworks.com

Fresh Sugar Lip Treatment, $22.50; Sephora, 877-737-4672 or sephora.com; fresh.com

Kiehl's Lip Balm #1, $5.50; kiehls.com

Laura Mercier Lip Silk, $20; Neiman Marcus, 888-888-4757; lauramercier.com

LIP LINER
Chanel Le Crayon Lèvres Precision Lip Definer in Tawny, $28; Neiman Marcus, 888-888-4757; chanel.com

MAC Cremestick Liner in Cream O' Spice, $14; MAC, 800-387-6707 or maccosmetics.com

LIPSTICK
Benefit Color Plump, $22; Sephora, 877-737-4672 or sephora.com; benefitcosmetics.com

Chanel Aqualumière Sheer Colour Lipshine SPF 15 in Waikiki, $25; Neiman Marcus, 888-888-4757; chanel.com

Clé de Peau Beauté Lipstick in 12, $55; Saks, 877-551-7257; Neiman Marcus, 888-888-4757

Clinique Long Last Soft Shine Lipstick in Bamboo Pink, $14; Bloomingdale's, 800-555-7467; clinique.com

Laura Mercier Lip Colour in Pink Champagne, $20; Saks, 877-551-7257; lauramercier.com

Yves Saint Laurent Rouge Pure Shine Sheer Lipstick #17 in Starlet Pink and #12 in Aqua Rose, $28; Saks, 877-551-7257; Nordstrom, nordstrom.com

LIP GLOSS
Chanel Lèvres Scintillantes Glossimer in Rose Sand, $25; Neiman Marcus, 888-888-4757; chanel.com

L'Oréal Paris Color Riche Lip Gloss in Soft Pink, $7.99; drugstores and mass retailers

MAC Tinted Lipglass in Prrr, $14; MAC, 800-387-6707 or maccosmetics.com

LIP LINE FILLERS
Patricia Wexler M.D. Dermatology Fastscription No-Injection Instant Line Filler for Lips and Eyes, $17.50; Bath & Body Works, 800-756-5005 or bathandbodyworks.com

LIP PLUMPERS
FusionBeauty LipFusion XL, $50; Sephora, 877-737-4672 or sephora.com

Patricia Wexler M.D. Dermatology Advanced Fastscription No-Injection Lip Plumper, $17.50; Bath & Body Works, 800-756-5005 or bathandbodyworks.com

FACIAL HAIR REMOVERS
Lineance Facial Hair Removal Cream, $12.99; drugstores and mass retailers

Parissa Strip Free Hot Wax, $9; parissa.com

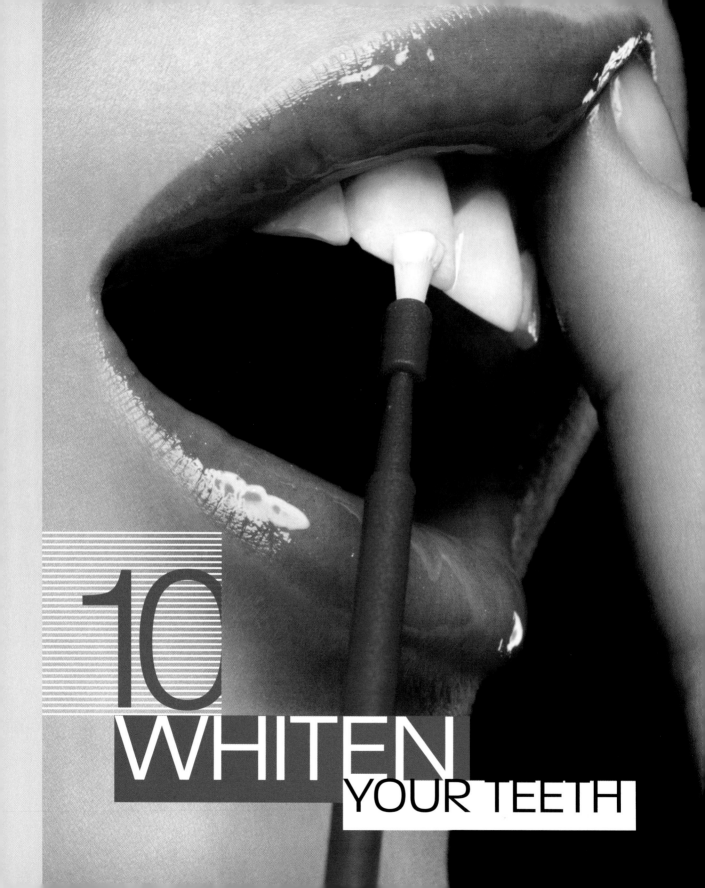

10

WHITEN
YOUR TEETH

NOTHING AGES YOU LIKE...
YELLOW TEETH... GRAY TEETH... STAINED OR SPLOTCHY TEETH... SMALL TEETH... RECEDING GUMS... TEETH THAT ARE TOO STRAIGHT ACROSS... A MOUTHFUL OF SILVER FILLINGS

What's sexier than flashing a big, white, movie-star smile? The operative words here are "big" and "white." It instant-messages the world: "I'm happy, healthy, vital, confident, and very much in the game, thank you!" You want to flash a big, sexy smile as much as you can (without looking like a Stepford wife) because a smile lifts your whole face upward — and that, as you know, is the direction we're heading in this book. What's OL is when an otherwise chic, sophisticated woman cups her hand over her mouth whenever she laughs, attempting to cover up embarrassing teeth. How sad to have to put on the brakes at those moments in life when you could be screaming with laughter!

Sorry to report that people are constantly making judgments about us — our upbringing, our education, our social status, our health — all based on the color, size, shape, and fit of our teeth. In fact, years ago, for the Broadway musical *Big River,* cosmetic dentist to the stars Dr. Jeff Golub-Evans fitted cast members who had dazzling actor smiles with snap-on "ugly teeth." These teeth were mismatched, ill shaped, overlapping, or spaced too far apart, in shades of dingy yellow and gray, to resemble those more befitting Huck Finn and his backwoods posse.

The good news is that no one who can afford it has to suffer from ugly teeth syndrome anymore. If you haven't had the good fortune to inherit a great set of choppers, you can buy them. It's the American way. And if you have great teeth but they have lost their brightness and whiteness over the years (as they tend to do), you can get them bleached. I don't understand why some women think nothing of dropping big bucks on, say, liposuction but blanch at investing money in cosmetic dental work. This doesn't make any sense. People see our teeth every waking hour; not as many see that tiny intersection of our butts and our thighs (unless we're in adult entertainment). So let's get our priorities straight. A great smile is a must-have if you want to look ten years younger.

This chapter is all about shopping for a killer smile, because you just can't be Y&H without it. "A great smile has become a fashion statement," says Dr. Golub-Evans, who has had Kim Cattrall, Usher, Hugh Jackman, and Regis Philbin in his chair at his New York Center for Cosmetic Dentistry on the Upper East Side of Manhattan. The fashion of the moment is a toothy grin that stretches from ear to ear, with beautifully shaped and polished teeth filling up every visible opening in your mouth. The quest for this movie-star smile has become a national obsession over the past decade. Cosmetic dentists report that women come armed with pages ripped from magazines, in hopes of replicating one of the most coveted smiles: Julia Roberts, Halle Berry, Gwyneth Paltrow, Heather Locklear, or, more recently, Jessica Simpson or Scarlett Johansson. (Is it any coincidence that Hollywood's most beautiful also have the most beautiful smiles?) This quest has changed our whole notion of going to the dentist. A dental appointment used to be anticipated with dread. Now it's more about getting gorgeous than filling cavities — just another appointment on the maintenance to-do list, along with haircut, hair color, and manicure. Dentistry has become so aesthetically focused that many have renamed their practices, and 5 percent of the dentists who belong to the American Dental Association (ADA) have gone so far as to reclassify their offices as spas (offering amenities such as pedicures, manicures, and facials). Wouldn't you rather go to the smile center, smile gym, or dental spa? We actually *want* to go to the dentist now. In fact, we've reached the point where we're seeing our dentists for checkups even more often than twice a year.

Getting back to Julia Roberts, Halle Berry, Gwyneth Paltrow, Heather Locklear, Jessica Simpson, and Scarlett Johansson . . . It doesn't matter whether their teeth are naturally theirs or charged on their credit cards. All that matters is that when they smile, they light up the room. So let's go to the dentist!

SHOPPING FOR A WHOLE NEW SMILE

For some, cosmetic dentistry is a way to address problems that should have been corrected years ago. That was the case with me. Everyone wore braces in junior high, but I didn't need them back then. When I left for college, however, my mouth got crowded, and one tooth started overlapping another. It was not a pretty sight, but no way

would I ever have considered having a metal mouth on campus. When I moved to New York City and started working at *Glamour* magazine, my teeth were discolored and jumbled. After work one day, while I was trying to catch a cab in front of the Condé Nast building, a *Glamour* editor, returning from a beauty shoot about smile styles (how to create a sexy, sophisticated, or sporty smile with bonding), offered me a ride. I climbed in, and Dr. Golub-Evans, who had supervised the shoot, took one look at my mouth and said, "It would be my greatest challenge to fix your teeth." Talk about a flattering pickup line! I laughed and replied, "I'll call you when I'm ready." I thought about it the next day, and the next day, and the next day. Booking that appointment was one of the best things I ever did for myself. For the first time in my life, I had a sexy smile — and I don't know how I could have ever had a TV career without it. In the mid-nineties, bonding was state-of-the-art. I've since graduated to porcelain veneers (details to come). The point of the story is, if I can have big, white, perfect teeth, so can you!

Even if you did have braces as a kid, your teeth may need a makeover due to normal wear and tear. As we age, our teeth tend to appear longer if our gums recede. That's the origin of the expression "She's a little long in the tooth." We hear it all the time in the magazine world, mostly in the context of, "Isn't that actress too old to be on the cover?" On the flip side, after years of grinding their teeth, some people wear down the enamel, so their teeth are shorter than they used to be or uniform in size all the way across. This is an OL look. You'll look younger if your two front teeth are longer than the teeth on either side. Whether your teeth are too long or too short; crooked, chipped, or overcrowded, your cosmetic dentist can create your new perfect smile — and with all the options available now, it probably won't be as much of a challenge as it was creating mine. Just make sure that your dentist uses the least invasive process to get the job done. Dr. Robert Schwartz, a respected dentist in Manhattan, says, "If I can barely touch someone's tooth, I'm thrilled. It's almost a crime to drill teeth that don't need to be drilled." The last thing you want to do is traumatize and file down a perfectly healthy, presentable tooth. So here are three options to keep you smiling, from least to most invasive.

Invisalign

If your teeth are merely crooked, you are a good candidate for these "adult braces," which are not nearly as embarrassing as they sound. More like trays than braces, they are almost undetectable to other people. When a friend of mine was wearing these, I wouldn't have known it if she hadn't told me. A dentist or orthodontist makes an impression of your teeth and then gives you a clear mold to wear. You wear it at all times except when eating, drinking, and brushing. The mold gently shifts your teeth. Every two weeks, you get a new mold that moves the teeth a little bit further, just as preteens visit the orthodontist to have their braces tightened every few weeks.

Upside: Your teeth aren't traumatized by any drilling. They remain your teeth.

Downside: The entire process takes a year and costs $4,500 to $8,000.

Bonding

If you have only a few teeth to fix, you can get away with bonding. It's ideal for lengthening or widening teeth, fixing chips, and making gaps between teeth disappear. A soft, pliable resin material is painted onto your existing tooth, then sculpted, filed, and polished to perfection. The

---

The White Teeth "Diet": Keeping Your Expensive Pearly Whites Pearly and White

Once you've labored to get your teeth to sparkle, protect your investment. Limit your intake of dark foods and drinks — such as blueberries, raspberries, black coffee, tea, red wine, and cranberry juice — as well as cigarettes (for a million and one health and beauty reasons). These can send your teeth right back to dullsville. If you can't wean yourself off coffee, add skim milk and sip it through a straw. Dr. Golub-Evans created "the White Teeth Diet." Here are some of his ways to navigate around the foods you love.

If you love:	Substitute:
Dark cola	Sprite or ginger ale
Dark tea	Light-colored tea
Red wine	Rosé, white wine, or champagne
Marinara sauce	Cream or clam sauce
Grape juice	White grape juice
Beets	Spinach, broccoli, or cauliflower
Cranberry juice	Grapefruit juice
Blueberries	Green grapes, apples, or raw carrots

And if you need more reasons to eat raw vegetables such as cucumbers and celery, you'll be happy to learn that they scrub away stains.

STAR STYLES
The Smiles Everyone Asks Her Cosmetic Dentist For

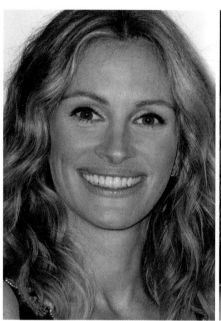

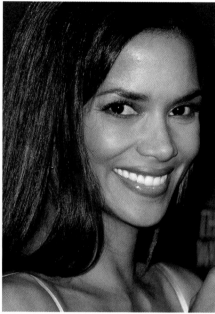

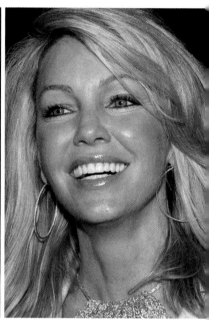

Julia Roberts   **Halle Berry**   **Heather Locklear**

resin mimics the color and consistency of tooth enamel, so it may be worth covering badly stained or discolored teeth with bonding if traditional whitening isn't working wonders. If teeth are poorly shaped or crooked, the bonding composite can be applied to an entire tooth.

Upside: Bonding is a relative bargain compared to porcelain veneers. At $300 to $500 per tooth, you're looking at $3,000 to $5,000 for ten teeth.

Downside: It lasts only three to five years, and bonding material is porous, so you have to watch out for stains — blueberries as well as red wine.

Porcelain Veneers
The choice of the high-maintenance woman. Pricey, yes, but they can give you that dazzling movie-star smile and cover all manner of sins, including teeth that are missing, overlapped, jagged, jumbled, chipped, crooked, worn down, or badly stained. Did we miss anything? Veneers won't! If you have ugly teeth and you never want to see them again, kiss them good-bye for the next twenty years with veneers.

Veneers are state-of-the-art dentistry. Not only is porcelain smoother, stronger, and longer lasting than bonding, but the glow it casts in your mouth is almost pearlescent, because the translucency of porcelain reflects light in a very realistic way. It's also highly resistant to stains, which polish off quickly, so you won't need additional whitening.

Getting veneers is a two-visit ordeal, two weeks apart. If your teeth are protruding out to "there," they unfortunately will need to be filed down so that when the porcelain shell is secured onto your existing tooth with a high-intensity light (it's almost like gluing on a fake nail), you won't look like Bucky Beaver. That said, this is the moment to speak up if you want a lip plump. One of the extra benefits of creating a new smile is that your dentist can "build out" your upper teeth, and fuller teeth push out your lips. (So much more effective than a tube of lip plumper!) After your first visit, you walk out with temporary teeth — a preview in bonding — so that you can get used to your new smile and test-drive the shape, style, size, fit, and color before getting the veneers (which are created in a lab off the premises, from a mold your dentist took).

If you love the look of veneers but not the drill-down, you'll be happy to know that the newest generation of ultrathin veneers don't require drilling. Although Dr. Schwartz has done hundreds of these, not everyone is a candidate. Your teeth cannot be too bulky; in this case, worn down or pulled back is a good thing.

To save money, you can get veneers on fewer teeth and cheat with bonding on those hard-to-see molars. Or do the top first and the bottom later, as I did. I've since learned from Dr. Schwartz, though, that's not the best strategy. Mismatched uppers and lowers don't look as glam as a matched set. But more than aesthetics, you're mismatching materials. Porcelain is stronger than enamel, so if you grind your teeth, the porcelain will win out, and the enamel will get worn down. Better to do it all at once if you can swing it financially.

| **Upside:** Unless you're opening beer bottles with them, veneers can last up to twenty-two years. And you don't have to worry about whitening anymore. | **Downside:** At a cost of $900 to $2,000 per tooth, ten teeth will set you back anywhere from $9,000 to $20,000 — amortized over twenty-two years! |

SHOPPING FOR THE RIGHT WHITE

"We live in a wonderful age when everyone can have white teeth," says Dr. Golub-Evans, talking about the fact that at just $25, the original Crest Whitestrips are priced to sell. PS: Every dentist I talk to says that Crest Whitestrips will get your teeth just as white as fancy in-office whitening treatments. Even so, whitening is by far the most requested procedure in cosmetic dentistry today. More than 100 million Americans whiten their teeth one way or another. It's predicted that this $600 million a year industry will reach $15 billion by the year 2010. Tooth whitening has become such an American obsession that we now have "bleacha-holics," men and women who simply can't curb their urge to go white, whiter, and whitest (not a good thing; more about that later). The truth is, the bar on what is the right white has been raised. Five years ago, what was beyond the range of normal white is now normal. In fact, all the composite bonding companies have had to make new shades because our teeth are so much whiter now. So if you haven't had your teeth whitened in the last five years, consider hitting the bleach.

How to Tell If You Should Hit the Bleach

OL teeth are dark, dingy, stained, yellow, or gray. Y&H teeth are white and bright. Don't let your teeth give your age away. The life we've lived shows on our teeth. Tooth enamel is so porous that a steady diet of coffee and colas can wreak damage over a lifetime. And think of all those dark-colored foods you love, from marinara sauce to chocolate, seeping into your pores and staining your enamel. When you don't brush your teeth at bedtime, you're practically inviting all those colors to get cozy on your pearly whites and settle in for the next eight hours. So if your teeth have yel-lowed (become dull or discolored from outside buildup), you have three relatively easy whitening options. But if your teeth are grayish (have become discolored internally, due to medication, trauma, or illness), don't waste your time and money on bleaching; go whiter with bonding or veneers instead. How to know if you're yellow or gray? Take the white paper test. Hold a sheet of white paper next to your teeth. Do your teeth look yellow or gray in comparison? Can't really tell? See your dentist.

Other Tooth To-Dos

✔ **Swear Off Lemon**
You want to protect your own tooth enamel as long as possible. Acidic foods, particularly lemons, can eat away at the enamel, exposing the dark tissue known as dentin underneath and making teeth look gray. You definitely don't want to suck on any lemons.

✔ **Use a Soft Tooth-brush**
A hard toothbrush seems like a good idea because it will help scrape off stains or buildup, but actually, you want to go soft. Hard toothbrushes are too abrasive and can erode the enamel. Choose a soft toothbrush and change it every three to four months (more often if you have had a cold, as the bristles can trap bacteria).

✔ **Keep On Brushing**
Did you know that you're supposed to brush your teeth for two minutes? Full disclosure: Until I started researching this, I didn't realize that my Sonicare electric toothbrush is programmed to shut off after two minutes — because I never kept it on for more than thirty seconds.

✔ **Floss**
Did you know that flossing could help you live longer? Aside from helping remove gunk between your teeth and gums, staving off the dreaded gum recession, studies show that people who floss have a lower incidence of heart disease. Yet only about 10 percent of Americans floss.

✔ **Get Professional Help**
Every three months may seem like a lot, but it's the recommended time for teeth cleaning and plaque removal with a dental hygienist. Schedule a cleaning before a big event so that your teeth sparkle from a professional polish.

✔ **Lose the Silver**
It's been many years since cavities were filled with silver, so if people spot the metal in your mouth, they'll know you've been around a while. Not to mention that silver is so distracting in contrast to your newly white teeth. Florida dentist Dr. Martin Polin says he wouldn't replace silver fillings merely for cosmetic reasons — the chances of hurting the tooth are too great — but if you have to replace fillings for another reason, by all means go white. Even Julia Roberts, poster girl for best smile, has silver fillings. When she was photographed at a red-carpet event with her mouth open wide, two celebrity magazines actually Photoshopped her silver fillings to make them white. If only we could do that in real life!

HIGH, MEDIUM, LOW MAINTENANCE . . . YOUR WHITEST SMILE

These three whitening treatments can all get you to the same level of white. So what do you have more of — money or time?

HIGH: In-office whitening is instant gratification. And like almost everything in life, it will cost you. Sometimes called chairside bleaching, it's the easiest, fastest, and most expensive route to a dazzling smile. All you have to do is sit back and relax for a couple of hours while someone else does all the work. Your dentist or hygienist will mask your gums to protect them from exposure to the bleaching gel, which contains a powerful dose of the potentially irritating hydrogen peroxide that's about to be painted onto your teeth. For twenty minutes, your teeth get hit with a light. Manufacturers claim that the light facilitates the bleaching action, but some dentists aren't convinced that it's anything more than marketing hype. Three or four rounds later, your teeth could be up to ten shades whiter. They'll be their absolute whitest when you leave the office — but don't get *too* excited, because they'll gradually fade a bit. That's why many dentists supply at-home touch-up trays so that you can follow up for one or two days three months later. And don't get upset if you need two or three in-office sessions to get your desired results — that's often the case. Depending on the staining power of the foods you eat and your diligence in brushing and flossing, you may need to revisit the in-office process yearly.

Going retail for this treatment is another option. Brite Smile, for instance, performs the same procedure and may charge less than your dentist. All things being relatively equal, it's preferable to go to your own dentist, who may pick up on something else at the same time. The technician at a retail outlet doesn't know you or your dental history regarding restorations (which won't be lightened by bleaching). Should anything go wrong, you're in the hands of "the dentist on the premises" — whoever that may be.

Upside: Speed, instant gratification, and you don't have to sleep with sloppy trays.

Downside: In-office whitening costs $500 to $1,200. And you may need to do it yearly.

MEDIUM: Custom whitening trays from your dentist are popular because they are less expensive than in-office whitening; they cost $350 to $900. The trade-off is that they take longer to work, which could cause gum sensitivity. First, your dentist will make a mold of your mouth. From this, she or he will create trays tailored precisely to fit your teeth and give you a tube of gel similar to the one used in chairside whitening. At home, you fill the trays with the solution, then stick them in your mouth from anywhere from half an hour to overnight for a period of two weeks. (These times vary depending on the percentage of peroxide in the gel, so you need to follow the instructions.)

Upside: When you need a touch-up, you don't have to go back to your dentist. Just pop in the trays for a few nights.

Downside: There's no one to monitor you. A bleachaholic with a whitening tray is like a foodaholic in the Cake of the Month Club. And wearing a tray overnight in bed isn't exactly sexy.

(PLEASE DON'T . . .)

Waste your money on trays sold in drugstores. One size does not fit all, so these trays are not going to be effective.

LOW: Crest Whitestrips Premium. If used correctly and consistently, they work as well as in-office or tray bleaching. There are several incarnations now, but with the Premium, you start to see results in less time — just three days. Wear the strips for thirty minutes twice a day and see full results in a week. The follow-up, Crest Whitestrips Renewal, claims to remove up to twenty years of stains in ten days. Each strip has a premeasured dose of peroxide, so you don't have to calculate how much to use.

Upside: Price ($34.99 for the Premium and $39.99 for the Renewal) and accessibility.	**Downside:** The strips are long enough to cover only the front six teeth.

$ Is It Worth It?

Whitening Products. Dentists say that in order for a bleaching solution to have any effect, it has to be in contact with the tooth for at least twenty minutes. So as you stroll down the drugstore aisle and see all those toothpastes, mouthwashes, gums, flosses, and mints that promise "whitening," be a smart shopper and save your money. All these products may be pleasant to use and give you sweet-smelling breath, but they're not penetrating deeply enough to change your color, though some do remove stains. "It's a gimmick, and it's more expensive," says Dr. Martin Polin, a cosmetic dentist who practices in Boca Raton, Florida. Dr. Polin would rather have you buy toothpaste with fluoride, because as your teeth recede, exposed roots can become more susceptible to cavities. But you didn't really think that whitening would be as easy as chewing gum anyway, did you?

How White Is Too White?

When I was handed a set of what looked like porcelain paint chips and asked to choose my shade, of course I pointed to the whitest. Fortunately, my dentist convinced me that "refrigerator white, aka Wayne Newton white," is not youthful-looking. Even though your teeth may be fake, you don't want them to *look* fake. Of course, some women love looking obvious. Dr. Polin says that many of his Boca Raton patients tell him, "I don't want to look natural. I have fake boobs; I want fake teeth!" In my opinion, there *is* such a thing as too white. The goal is to have your teeth look real, not like Chiclets. The reaction you're going for is, "Wow, what a great smile," not "Wow, your teeth are really white." So when you're asked to choose your dream white, listen to your dentist and back up a shade or two. If you're using at-home trays or Crest Whitestrips, stop if you think you're getting too white. Too white is OL. You don't want to look like a used-car salesman!

(PLEASE DON'T . . .)

Become a bleachaholic. The process, no matter where it's performed, was not meant to be done daily. Chronic whitening can cause hypersensitivity to cold and heat, which is not something you want.

The Good Gums Diet

Chances are you already analyze everything you eat, judging each morsel for its calories, fat grams, dietary fiber, calcium quotient, effect on cholesterol, and so on. Now you can add one more consideration: How will your dinner affect your gums? If you are already meticulous about brushing, flossing, and getting regular checkups, eat whatever your heart desires; you deserve it! But for the rest of us, who are not exemplars of oral hygiene rectitude, it's good to know not only those foods that keep teeth white (as we already covered) but also those that naturally keep our gums pink, healthy, and plaque-free. Rinsing with water for twenty seconds immediately after downing anything on the "bad" list will help. When I went to see Dr. James Jacobs, a New York City periodontist, he regaled me with a list of what's good and bad for gums.

Good for the Gums

■ Fibrous fruits and raw vegetables — such as apples, pears, peaches, plums, celery, carrots, cucumbers, pickles, broccoli, asparagus, grapes, green beans, mushrooms, and bananas — act like a detergent, cleaning the surfaces of your teeth as you chew.

■ Oranges, pineapples, grapefruits, tangerines, nectarines, honeydews, cantaloupes, limes, mangoes, and tomatoes have a lot of vitamin C, which is good for gum tissue. Lemons, though also high in vitamin C, are too acidic for tooth enamel.

Bad for the Gums

■ Sticky foods such as taffy and caramel, which get stuck in your teeth.

■ Plaque magnets such as cheese and chocolate.

■ Sugary foods such as white bread, cookies, doughnuts, and muffins. They hang out in your mouth longer than they should and get stickier as they go through the digestive tract.

■ Popcorn — the chief bête noire of dentists everywhere. All too often, kernels get lodged between teeth or slide under the gums, where they can cause an abscess.

B R I L L I A N T   B U Y S

TOOTHPASTE
Crest Pro-Health Toothpaste, $4.49; drugstores and mass retailers
Colgate Total Toothpaste, $3.59; drugstores and mass retailers

TOOTHBRUSH
Philips Sonicare FlexCare, $179.99; Target, 800-440-0680; amazon.com

MOUTHWASH
ACT Anticavity Fluoride Rinse (alcohol-free; 18 ounces), $5.29; Target, 800-440-0680; drugstore.com
Crest Pro-Health Rinse, $5.29; drugstores and mass retailers

WHITENING
Crest Whitestrips Premium, $34.99; drugstores and mass retailers
Crest Whitestrips Renewal, $39.99; Target, 800-440-0680; drugstore.com

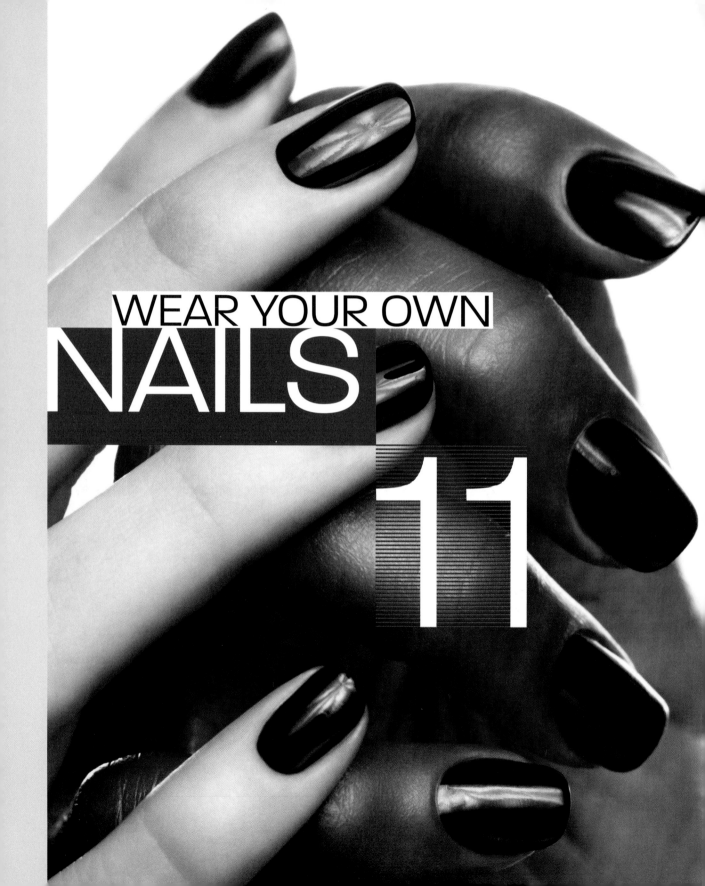

WEAR YOUR OWN
NAILS

11

NOTHING AGES YOU LIKE...
RED NAIL POLISH... FAKE NAILS... DRAGON-LADY NAILS... RIDGED NAILS... DISCOLORED NAILS... AGE SPOTS ON YOUR HANDS... VEINY HANDS... BONY HANDS

In the fall of 2006, the hottest nail polish color in the country was Black Satin by Chanel. The inky, dark-as-doom varnish generated waiting lists at department stores, was listed on eBay for $50 a bottle, and spawned tons of imitations. The dark-polish fad (and it resurges every few years) presents women over twenty-five with a quandary: Do you paint your nails black and mark yourself as trendy and knowing, or do you do everything in your power to deflect attention from your hands? It depends on how happy you are with the look of your hands. If they're soft and pretty, show them off with dark polish. But if you haven't been pampering your hands all these years (and unless you're a hand model, I'm guessing you haven't), by all means deflect! You may have naturally luminous skin or a regular date with a vial of Botox that lets your face lie about its age, but your hands will always give you away. Chances are they reveal one or two telltale OL signs, whether it's brown spots, visible veins, red spots, or protruding bones. If you're super high maintenance, you might consider lasers or injections for hand imperfections (more on these later in this chapter), but for the rest of us, it's best not to draw attention to this part of your body when you can easily have people looking elsewhere.

The most important factor in making your hands unobtrusive is the look of your nails. Keep them short, neat, clean, and painted in a neutral color. That way, your hands will look natural and healthy. Not only are long, dragon-lady nails scary

(think Cruella de Vil), tacky (think Carmela Soprano), and OL (think your mother), but they also can make it a challenge to use a computer, text-message, call from a cell phone, or do just about anything else a modern woman needs to do. Just FYI, you already know that nails should be well manicured, never chipped or jagged, but it's this finishing touch to your overall Y&H look that shows that you take care of yourself and pay attention to every last detail.

DON'T GET NAILED
A lot of women spend a lot of money to get artificial nails. I say, don't bother! Liberate yourself from the glue, the smell, and the expense. This is one of those cases where the cover-up is worse than the problem. Many upscale salons don't even offer them anymore. (If you needed to fix an artificial nail in Manhattan, it would be a challenge to find a salon that could handle it.) Now, I realize that although discussing faux nails is not like discussing politics or religion, opinions on them can be polarizing. In certain parts of the country, they're considered a beauty birthright, and every time I've been on television or written an article urging women to "Just Say No" to them, I've gotten calls and letters from the Nail Industrial Complex — those who supply and apply artificial nails. But I'm not going to lie to you: long faux nails just aren't Y&H. What's more, they increase the likelihood of your getting a fungus under your nails, which could lead to an infection. Another argument for keeping nails real is that

Take Time off Your Hands

Our hands get as much exposure to the elements as our faces, but do we slather them with SPF 30 daily? Not many of us do. Here are some simple, fast things to get your hands looking better.

■ Apply sunscreen to them every morning and reapply it throughout the day.

■ Get a weekly manicure.

■ Wear rubber gloves every time you do the dishes.

■ Moisturize your hands every time they come in contact with water.

■ Never use your nails as a "tool" to open cans, letters, or boxes; peel off stickers; or perform other tasks.

■ Before bed, slather on Vaseline or a thick moisturizer, then slip on a pair of cotton or rubber-lined gloves.

■ Rub on cuticle oil every morning and night.

■ When you get a manicure, bring your own tool kit, to avoid any chance of infection. (This one is a must.)

---

you can actually see the condition of your nails and know if they are peeling, weak, ridged, discolored, and so on. If your nails suffer any of these ills, it's always better to fix the problem than mask it. Take a stroll down the drugstore nail care aisle, where you'll find a paint-on solution for every problem (see Brilliant Buys).

Y&H NAIL TIPS

A few pointers for keeping your fingertips looking terrific, whether you get a professional manicure or do it yourself.

■ **Shape:** It's been around for years and it's still as chic as ever: "squoval." Not quite square and not quite oval, this is the flattering shape in between. It's the ideal form for a natural-looking nail.

■ **Length:** Keep nails no longer than a quarter inch beyond your fingertips, which is to say, ever so slightly longer than your finger.

■ **Color:** Don't get me wrong, I love fun, outrageous nail polish colors, but I usually save them for my toes. On fingernails, a pretty, sheer pink or beige will take you anywhere, from a business lunch to a wedding. Light colors elongate the look of your fingers, whereas bright colors can make them look stubby. Another downside to vivid colors is that they are incredibly tough to maintain. If you're wearing nail polish and you dare to open an envelope or wash a dish, you can easily chip your polish. A nick is much more obvious with a dark polish than with a sheer one — and so much more difficult to fix. For starters, you need the exact same shade. Sheers all blend into each other, and you're pretty sure to have a sheer around the house, in the car, at the office, or in your bag.

The French manicure can be tricky (and look OL) if not done right. If you can't wean yourself away, follow the suggestion of celebrity manicurist Deborah Lippmann, who manicures Reese Witherspoon, Mary J. Blige, and Kate Winslet, among others: "The French manicure should be a soft white, not a stark white, . . . and the tip should be applied very thin. Nine times out of ten, it's too thick, which makes it not chic."

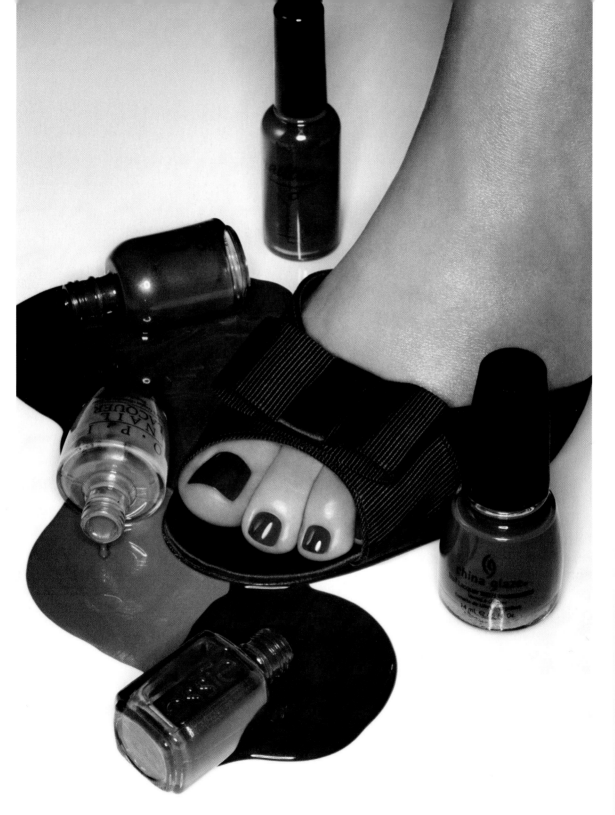

Go wild on your tootsies.

(PLEASE DON'T . . .) Even think about nail art. There is nothing classy about rhinestones, appliqués, decals, or multicolored polish. Also, avoid anything with excessive glitter. It will make you look like you crashed a sleepover party.

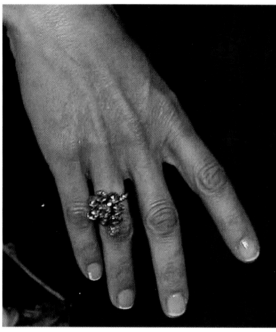

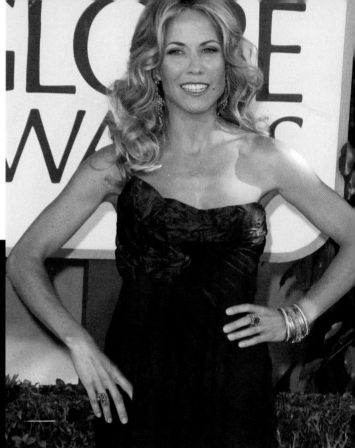

JUST RIGHT: Sheryl Crow's short, light, natural nails, even for evening

The Newer Way to . . .
Do Faux Nails

If you absolutely, positively insist on having long nails, forgo traditional acrylics and check out the Custom Blended Manicure by Creative Nail Design. The process, which starts at $55, was created to help nails grow long, so there's no need to apply artificial nails. At salons where it's done (you can

find one at creativenaildesign.com), a professional manicurist blends pigmented powders to create a resin coating that matches the color of your nails. The coating fortifies nails so they won't split, peel, chip, or break. It only requires upkeep every three weeks and looks very real. I featured these nails on the *Today* show, and the model, who had terrible-looking nails beforehand, was thrilled.

$ Is It Worth It?

Paraffin Treatments. You may be spending time and money on paraffin treatments either at the salon, the spa, or at home. Yes, the hot wax and gloves make your paws feel fabulously soft, but they won't erase the years. Dr. Neil Sadick, a pioneer in the rejuvenation of hands, says, "It's just pampering."

HIGH AND LOW MAINTENANCE . . .
ANTIAGING YOUR HANDS

If weekly manicures and prodigious amounts of lotion don't take nine years off your hands, it may be time to ramp up your strategy. When it comes to hands, there really isn't much of a medium-maintenance option, but stay tuned.

HIGH: What a dermatologist can do for your face, he or she also can do for your hands. Dr. Sadick suggests that to prevent damage, you can start having light peels and laser work in your forties. In your fifties, you may need to start using fillers. Popular laser treatments for hands include intense pulsed light (IPL), which uses light to target brown sun spots (aka age spots or liver spots, which is about the most OL-sounding thing I've ever heard). After treatment, the zapped spots dry up and peel off. To make sure they don't return, you must keep your hands well protected from the sun. A more drastic option is the Fraxel laser, which stimulates collagen under the skin and helps resurfacing (see chapter 8).

If your problem is ropy, knobby hands, look into fillers. The same substances that plump up lines in your face, can plump up your hands. As we age, our hands lose fullness, which makes everything under the skin protrude. Injectables such as Restylane and Sculptra are being used to fill in the areas around the veins and bones and make them appear less prominent. The results can last six months or longer. On the filler forefront, Dr. Sadick has developed laser fiber, the EVLH (Endovenous Laser), with the Cool Touch Corporation, which is inserted into the hand. It's preferable to fillers because you don't have to get your hands (who has time?) filled every six months (Restylane) or every couple of years (Sculptra). For $1,500 (both hands), you're done.

LOW: Apply retinol at night and an alpha hydroxy cream with sunscreen during the day to the skin on the back of your hands to improve texture and lighten dark patches. Just as with your face, though, results are slow in coming. If you're behind the wheel a lot during the day, driving gloves will protect your hands from further sun damage and can look quite chic.

B R I L L I A N T   B U Y S

NAIL CARE
Creative Nail Design Solar Oil (0.5 oz.), $9; Ulta Beauty Supply, 866-340-3704; goindulge.com
Lippmann Collection The Stripper Lavender Lacquer Remover, $16; Bath & Body Works, bathandbodyworks.com; lippmanncollection.com

NAIL COLOR
Essie Limo-scene, $8; essie.com for stores
Lippmann Collection Nail Lacquers, $15; Bath & Body Works, bathandbodyworks.com; lippmanncollection.com
L'Oréal Paris PRO Manicure, I Pink I'm in Love, $4.99; drugstores and mass retailers
OPI Lincoln Park After Dark, $8; OPI, 800-341-9999 for stores

HAND CREAM
Clarins Age-Control Hand Lotion SPF 15, $29; clarins.com
Prescriptives Intensive Rebuilding Hand Treatment SPF 15, $38; prescriptives.com

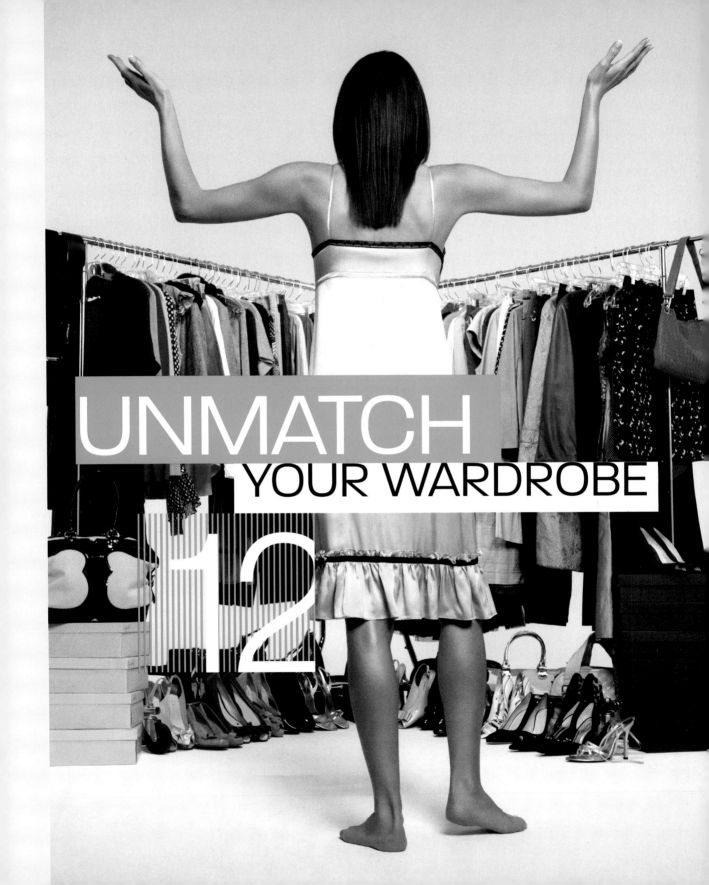

UNMATCH
YOUR WARDROBE

12

NOTHING AGES YOU LIKE . . .
OUTFITS THAT ARE TOO MATCHY-MATCHY . . . DRESSING HEAD TO TOE IN ONE DESIGNER . . . LOOKING LIKE YOU TRIED TOO HARD . . . LOOKING LIKE YOU DIDN'T TRY AT ALL . . . CLOTHES THAT ARE TOO YOUNG

If you walk down Madison Avenue in New York City or Michigan Avenue in Chicago and spot a woman dressed head to toe in a designer outfit with shoes and bag to match, you can bet that she's over sixty. She might look perfectly polished, but she doesn't look Y&H. Plunking down a credit card for the designated uniform of one designer is OL because it lacks personal style, big-time. It's as if you walked into someone's home and every piece of furniture, every accessory was bought in the same store and assembled exactly the way it looks in the catalog. Of course, there's nothing wrong with having your house look like a page ripped from the Pottery Barn catalog (and for some, I realize, it would be a dream come true). But we're talking you, and we're raising the bar. The truth is, it's not the modern way to dress. What's modern is an eclectic mix that celebrates your unique personal style. (Don't say, "What personal style?" You have one, even if you don't recognize it yet!) So get the concept of "complete outfit" out of your mind. Don't shop for head-to-toe outfits, and don't hang complete outfits in your closet. Instead, buy a fresh new piece that speaks to the current fashion moment, and make sure the color and style mix well with at least two pieces you already own.

To see all the possibilities in your closet, organize it in terms of color, piece by piece. For inspiration, go into a hip boutique, where you'll find the store organized by pieces, not outfits. It's now up to the shopper to mix and layer tops, jackets, and sweaters with pants, skirts, and jeans until she finds combinations that flatter her particular figure and zing with personal style. If you walk down the street and spot a woman wearing a black sweater coat cinched at the waist with a big, thick, patent leather belt; an animal-print pencil skirt; brown suede, knee-high boots; and an oversized yellow bag, well, that's Y&H. It's quirky, interesting, not cookie-cutter. It exudes the swingy, confident, independent spirit of someone who knows that the sweater coat is the new jacket, which will instantly update all the go-the-distance classics hanging in her closet. By the end of this chapter, you will have that spirit, too. You will have merchandised your own closet so that the outfits you create look effortlessly chic, as if you just threw them together. Effortlessly chic is Y&H. Trying too hard is OL. There is a delicate tipping point here, and you will master the art of looking as if you made an effort, but not *too* much of an effort!

DITCH THE OLD FASHION RULES AND PICK UP THE NEW ONES

Before you can embrace the new rules of fashion, you must erase the old ones from your memory. We're talking old rules such as "Match your shoes to your handbag and everything else," along with "Don't wear white after Labor Day." Making this change isn't easy, since the old rules have been on repeat play in your subconscious since you were sweet sixteen. But once you get the new rules, you'll find dozens of outfits in your closet you didn't know existed. And best of all, the new rules will actually save you money, because if you were to amortize your MVPs (most valuable pieces) over each time you wear them, you would be thrilled at how economical those buys turned out

to be. You will be buying less and wearing your clothes more when you follow the new rules. You will up the versatility of, say, your perfect white ruffled shirt, your black cashmere turtleneck, your brown straight skirt, and your dark denim jeans. Fashion insiders love to throw up their hands and announce, "There are no rules anymore!" But they're not being completely honest. Of course there are rules; there are new rules.

The Old Rules vs. The New Rules

Old	New
Always match your handbag to your shoes.	Matchy-matchy will make you look oldie-oldie.
Don't wear white after Labor Day.	Wear white in the winter and black in the summer — so chic!
Don't wear black and navy together.	Mix black with navy—and brown.
Don't wear different shades of black together.	Mix black with black whatever the tones.
Never mix two different prints or patterns in the same outfit.	Mixed patterns look fresh when matched according to color tones.
Metallic pieces are for evening only.	Metallics are for day, too. They're the new neutral.
Stockings should be flesh toned.	Shoes should be flesh toned, legs bare.
Don't wear costume jewelry.	Faux can be fabulous (just don't blab about it).
Jeans are for daytime only.	Jeans are hot and sexy for evening — with heels and an embellished top.

Y&H Effortlessly Chic **Wardrobe** Essentials

Build your wardrobe with these classic essentials. Invest in the best, and they will be part of your wardrobe for years:

- Black and white cashmere cardigans
- Black and white cashmere turtlenecks
- Cashmere V-neck sweaters in colors
- Fitted black leather jacket

- Fitted winter and summer jackets
- Silk T-shirts in black, white, and cream
- Delicate camisoles in black, white, and cream
- Crisp, white, ruffled blouse
- Black straight skirt

- Tailored trousers in black, brown, beige, and gray
- Black sheath dresses for winter and summer
- Dark denim jeans
- Fitted trench coat in a wow color or fabric

THE BASICS OF LOOKING EFFORTLESSLY CHIC

Okay, now we're set to get the scoop on Y&H dressing, shopping, and closet organizing that every fashionista follows but never talks about.

Get Casual: Loosen Up Your Look — but Only So Far

In today's workplace, every day has become Casual Friday. To me, it's not such a good thing. Some looks are not office appropriate for women of any age. They include super-low-riding jeans, ripped jeans, shoulder-baring halter dresses, midriff-baring tops, breast-baring camisoles, tight message T-shirts, microminis, hot pants, and flip-flops (the office is not the beach). But this has become the new norm for people who work in "creative fields," and you can see how a woman of a certain age wearing a designer skirt and matching jacket, stockings, and pumps would immediately signal OL on the premises. The modern way to dress is to look a little less "sprayed," as Sharyn Soleimani, personal shopper extraor-

dinaire at Barneys New York, puts it. "Dress less finished, and you'll look younger," she says. "When you're very young, you can be very finished and you still look young. But when you're more mature, imperfection looks so much better. For some women, it's very hard not to be perfect, not to have every hair in place, not to have too much makeup on!" Which is where Sharyn comes in. "For some women, I just tell them, 'If you're going to the movies, put this jacket with this pant. If you're going to the theater, wear the jacket with this little straight skirt and a sexy tank underneath.' For some people, I write it out on index cards!"

It's important to fight the desire to overdress, even outside the workplace. If you're going to a casual dinner party at a friend's home on a Saturday night in the summer, a skirt and matching jacket (even if it's by Chanel — and who doesn't love Chanel?) is too much. Ditch the suit and wear the jacket (or better, a cardigan) with white jeans and strappy sandals. The goal is to look casual, but appropriately casual. That translates into fewer suits and more separates put together in a fresh, unexpected way. This is the essence of looking effortlessly chic. Once you unleash yourself from the suit-as-uniform way of dressing, you will feel liberated and look ten years (or more!) younger.

TOO OLD: matchy-matchy

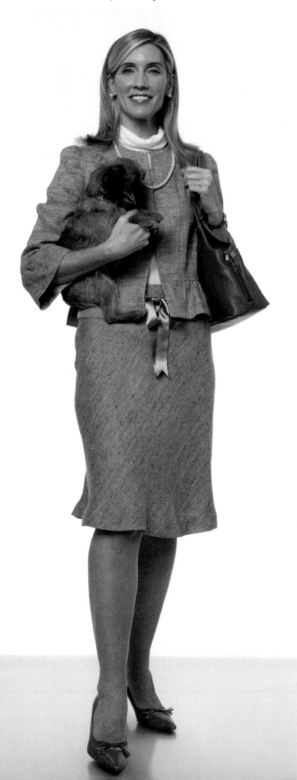

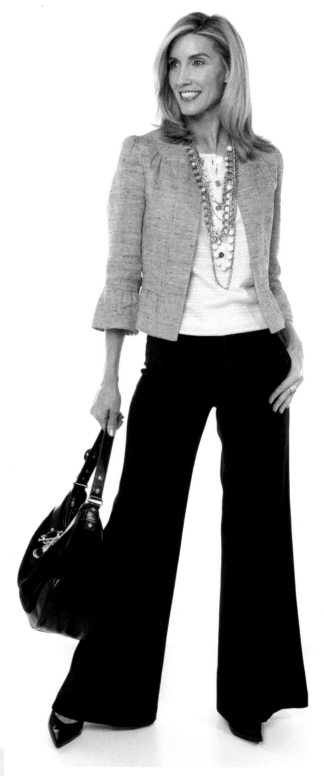

JUST RIGHT: take the same jacket, lose the skirt, add of-the-moment accessories, and you're Y&H.

Y&H Effortlessly Chic **Accessory** Essentials

- Gold hoop earrings
- Diamond stud earrings
- Classic watch with gold and silver chain links
- Chunky bangle bracelets
- Sleek black heels
- Sparkly evening clutch

- Quality leather bag for day
- Quality tote bag for books, magazines, and newspaper
- Nude heels
- Black and brown knee-high boots

- Black- and brown-heeled shoe booties
- Black, brown, navy, and gray opaque tights
- Black, brown, gold, and silver belts
- Chunky-chain necklace

Dress Fashionably, but Don't Be a Fashion Victim

There's a big difference between being a slave to the latest trends and being aware of them. You want the latter. Every season, the fashion industry presents hundreds of trends. Some are exciting, some are fun, some are silly, and some are downright idiotic. Your mission is to be a smart shopper and buy only the trends that work for you — your body, your personality, your lifestyle. Take your cues from the lists in this chapter — "Top 25 Clothes That Just Gotta Go" and "Too Young!" You want to dress appropriately Y&H — not with clothes that date you, and not with clothes that are designed with the twentysomething in mind. Picking up every hot trend is a little like going out with every guy you see; you have to be discriminating, or you will end up a mess. A fashion victim doesn't discriminate but rather desperately invests in all things trendy, whether or not they look good on her.

Each season, fashion coach Susan Sommers, whose business, DressZing, helps women shop in their closets, advises her clients to ask themselves, " 'What one or two pieces will make my wardrobe pop right now?' They don't have to be super-expensive, but they should be of the moment." If the of-the-moment piece is pricey, before you splurge, ask yourself, "Is this something I can wear after this season is over?" Treat your wardrobe as an art collection, and curate it with pieces that are worth

the investment because they go the distance. If you have doubts, skip it. Know that you can always add a hit of style with more disposable items, such as of-the-moment costume jewelry and other fun, instant-gratification accessories.

Learn to Love Classics — with a Twist

Dressing effortlessly chic makes great use of classic shapes. When stocking up, think cardigans, V-necks, sheaths, a peacoat, a trench coat. These classic shapes have been around since the invention of clothing, and to keep them from being, well, classically boring, make sure they have some kind of "a twist," as Sharyn Soleimani says. Maybe it's a cashmere cardigan without buttons. Maybe it's a V-neck in a fresh color. A trench coat in black patent leather, rather than the expected khaki, becomes edgy. Jacqueline Kennedy Onassis, who was the picture of ageless chic throughout her life, seldom strayed from the classics. A simple cashmere turtleneck sweater, a pretty twinset, a black sheath dress, fitted tweed trousers, and designer pumps kept her looking positively girlish — and effortlessly chic — well into her sixties. The idea of classic, casual shapes in quality fabrics holds true for every

Too Young!

Here's a list of forbidden fashion items for every woman past the age of thirty who wants to look effortlessly chic and classy.

Ankle bracelets	Earmuffs	Newsboy caps
Belly necklaces	Ear piercing in multiples	Scrunchies
Body piercing	Flip-flops in the city	Super-low-riding jeans
Boy shorts	Go-go boots	Tattoos
Collegiate sweats, T-shirts, and caps	Leg warmers	Tie-dye anything
Colored cowboy boots	Microminidresses	Tights in neon colors
Crocs (out of the garden)	Microminiskirts	Toe rings
Daisy dukes	Mittens	Tube tops
	Nameplate necklaces	(as stand-alones)

occasion — even fancy cocktail parties. The idea is to find classic shapes in dressier fabrics such as eyelet, silk, chiffon, brocade, or velvet when the occasion calls for something special.

Forgive me if I repeat myself, but I can't say this enough: No matter how classic the shape, and no matter how hot it may be right now, don't be tempted to wear anything that doesn't flatter you. The piece has to be in proportion for your body shape. The tunic, for example, is a classic shape that's in fashion right now, but if you're very petite, a long tunic can overwhelm you and make you look like a sack of potatoes. This is a hard, hard lesson to learn, but one worth repeating every time you're in the dressing room: *If it doesn't look good on you, it doesn't look good, period!* Which brings me to my most important shopping to-do . . .

Don't Buy It If You Don't Love It. And Love It Only If It Flatters You!

It doesn't matter what big name is on the label. It doesn't matter how low the price. Does the piece flatter you? Does it make you look thinner, younger, hipper? Does it make you feel powerful? That's what matters. The lesson here: Buy less, buy better, be picky. If you can walk away without getting a

pang, do yourself a favor and walk away. You don't need another piece of clothing in your closet taking up valuable real estate.

Dress Young, but Not Teenage Young

It's fine to shop for fun accessories and costume jewelry at stores such as Forever 21 and Claire's, but buying clothing at a retailer that caters to juniors will only make you look like an OL who is trying too hard to look Y&H. There's a reason that the prices are cheaper in the teen department. The fabrics are cheap! And cheap fabrics are never flattering, especially on women over seventeen.

Many of the mistakes that grown women make when trying to look young fall into the category of revealing too much, as in baring your midriff (unless you're at the beach). It doesn't matter if you have six-pack abs or paid six figures for a tummy tuck, keep it hidden — it's not cute!

HIGH, MEDIUM, AND LOW MAINTENANCE . . . EDITING YOUR CLOSET

By now you should have an idea that dressing Y&H is all about pieces, pieces, pieces! You also have some good basic guidelines to follow and the essential items to have on hand. Now it's time to edit your closet to reflect your new way of dressing. Separate by category (tops, blouses, dresses, jackets, skirts, pants, jeans). Don't even think about creating an outfit and putting it on the same hanger. That will take those pieces out of the running of getting paired with something much chicer. Muster up the courage to toss anything that is shabby, dirty, or stained; doesn't feel right; or has been sitting in the closet for more than two years collecting dust. Repeat this process for every season.

HIGH: Go ahead and hire a personal stylist to help edit your closet every season. This is not as extravagant as it seems. For less than what it costs to buy one new designer outfit, a savvy stylist can help you shop in your closet and create twenty or more outfits you never knew you had. This is a smart way to get more mileage out of what you already own. I do this every season. My friend Susan Sommers, the fashion coach, takes digital photos of the "new outfits" we've created and sends them to me. I print them out and staple them in a small book that I keep in my closet. Whenever I'm stumped for what to wear, I find the answer in my book.

There is nothing like a pair of professional eyes to advise you on what to keep, what to store, and what to donate. A professional is less likely to care about hurting your feelings than a friend and will be more inclined to lay down the law if something is terribly unflattering. Believe me, I know how emotionally attached one can get to clothes. Parting with longtime friends can be painful, but it's absolutely necessary to keep you looking Y&H. If you have designer clothes that don't look good on you anymore, the newer way to get rid of them is on eBay.

Top 25 Clothes That Just Gotta Go

No matter how attached you are to any of these pieces, it's time to part company, because they will date you and make you look OL. Don't even think about keeping them for stay-around-the-house days, as you don't want to be caught in them if the FedEx guy rings your bell. How fast can you get them out of your drawers and closets?

1. Holiday sweaters with bells and appliqués (reindeers, teddy bears, bumblebees, pumpkins)
2. Granny/mommy necklaces that tell how many grandchildren/children you have
3. Souvenir T-shirts
4. T-shirts with meant-to-be-funny sayings
5. Overalls
6. Acid-washed jeans
7. Ripped jeans
8. Shoulder pads
9. Flannel shirts
10. Muumuus
11. Photo handbags (no matter how cute the kids!)
12. Flesh-colored hose
13. Penny loafers
14. Oversized blazers
15. Mommy robes
16. Thin-gold-chain necklaces
17. Elastic-waist pants
18. Granny undies
19. Baggy sweats
20. Bearlike, full-length fur coats
21. Short shorts
22. Cargo pants
23. Stockings with reinforced toes
24. Three-piece suits with vests
25. Backpacks

(The old way is a consignment shop. But you really have to keep on top of this. It's your responsibility to check to see if the things you dropped off were sold.) If the clothes are not designer, donate them to charity and collect your tax deduction.

MEDIUM: Ask a friend to come over and have her weigh in as you try on everything in your closet. Ask her to be brutally honest. (You can do her the same favor.) Follow all the steps for low maintenance, but have her take the digital photos of you in your new hip outfits.

LOW: You're going to fly solo. Clear your calendar for the better part of a day. Try on all your clothes in front of a full-length mirror and analyze each item, asking yourself, "Does this make me look old?" and if not, "What can I wear this with?" Mix and match your pieces (including stockings, shoes, and jewelry). When you fall in love with a look, lay it out on your bed and take a digital picture.

BECOME A MIX MASTER

You've stocked up on classic shapes and purged your closet of everything that makes you look old or too young. You've let go of all those old rules about what to wear with what. But how do you mix pieces in a fresh, modern way so that they look Y&H?

Mix Prints: Four Secrets

Yes, you can mix prints, even if they're as different as florals and stripes.

1. Different prints, such as plaids, polka dots, florals, stripes, and houndstooth checks, can be mixed together. But under no circumstances can you mix different animal prints. Just one piece of leopard or zebra or giraffe per outfit, please!

2. You must have a unifying color palette within the prints.

3. To mix the same type of print — floral with floral, or houndstooth with houndstooth — they must be of drastically different scales.

4. There must be a solid piece somewhere in your outfit — T-shirt, shoes, jeans — to anchor the mixed prints.

Fashion designer Isaac Mizrahi's rule: "You have to try everything on. Everything with everything. So you can actually get a sense of what looks the rightest wrong. . . . Let's face it, looking a little off is as much work as looking on!"

Mix Designer and Nondesigner, or Luxe and Less

Sharon Stone made fashion history the day she paired a Vera Wang skirt with a black Gap T-shirt and wore it to the Oscars — and told the world that she just threw them together at the last minute! The press she got for being so clever was off the charts. French women have been doing the mix for years. When they wear classy black basics and toss in a fun plastic bracelet that they bought at Monoprix, no one is going to suspect that the bracelet cost 2 euros. That's because the rest of the package is presented so elegantly. Isaac Mizrahi won raves from the fashion crowd when years ago, he staged his first fashion show with models wearing sweaters from his Target line paired with couture ball gowns from his Bergdorf Goodman line. "One hard-and-fast rule for the past seven years or so and going into the future is that you can't wear all expensive clothes," he says. "You have to have something inexpensive on to democratize the whole thing!" This from a designer who offers an expensive line, too. So don't be a fashion snob. Wear that great-fitting T-shirt from Banana Republic under a Ralph Lauren jacket. It doesn't matter what it costs anymore; it just matters that it looks great on you. And there's never been a better time in the history of shopping to mix high and low. When stores such as Target, JCPenney, H&M, Kmart, Spiegel, and Kohl's are hiring big-name designers such as Mizrahi, Nicole Miller, Karl Lagerfeld, Stella McCartney, Norma Kamali, and Vera Wang, the shopper wins.

Here's a simple breakdown of ageless labels that are perfect for mixing. Just choose your price points: high, medium, or low.

HIGH

Chanel

Dolce & Gabbana

Donna Karan

Michael Kors

Prada

Ralph Lauren

MEDIUM

Banana Republic

Club Monaco

Milly

Tevrow & Chase

Theory

Tory Burch

LOW

H&M

Isaac Mizrahi for Target

Nicole Miller for JCPenney

Top Shop

Very Vera Wang by Vera Wang for Kohl's

Zara

DO YOU LOOK EFFORTLESSLY CHIC?

Before you walk out the door, take a minute to look in the mirror and ask yourself if you look effortlessly chic. If the answer is yes, you're outta there. If you hesitate at all, you've tried too hard, and trying too hard is one of the most common mistakes that can label you OL. You need to, as they say in the fashion biz, "take it down a notch."

The way to do this is by introducing a casual piece into the mix. For instance, if you're wearing a sequined tank and need a cover-up, consider a cropped cardigan rather than a rhinestone suit jacket. Another way to bring it down a notch is to change to a more casual shoe. Switch from a four-inch pump to an open-toe platform sandal. Here are some other ways to instantly take it down a notch.

- **Hoop earrings** instead of chandelier earrings
- **Beltless** rather than a flashy belt
- **A wedge** instead of a high-heeled sandal
- **A plain white T-shirt** instead of a lacy camisole
- **Dark denim jeans** instead of black trousers
- **White jeans** rather than white pants or a skirt
- **Earrings** instead of a jeweled necklace
- **Small diamond studs** rather than longer earrings

Remember, the look you're trying to achieve is effortlessly chic — not effortless! The flip side of looking like you've tried too hard is looking like you haven't tried at all. For example, showing up at the airport in sweats, sneakers, and a fanny pack looks just plain sloppy. There are chicer ways of dressing comfortably, such as dark denim jeans, a cashmere sweater, and sport shoes (see chapter 18). When you're traveling, avoid the dreaded OL tourist uniform: sneakers, baggy jeans, oversized T-shirt or sweatshirt, and fanny pack. Dress to look chic on the streets of whatever city you're in. And remember that the chicer you look, the better you'll be treated — in restaurants, in stores, in hotels, in line.

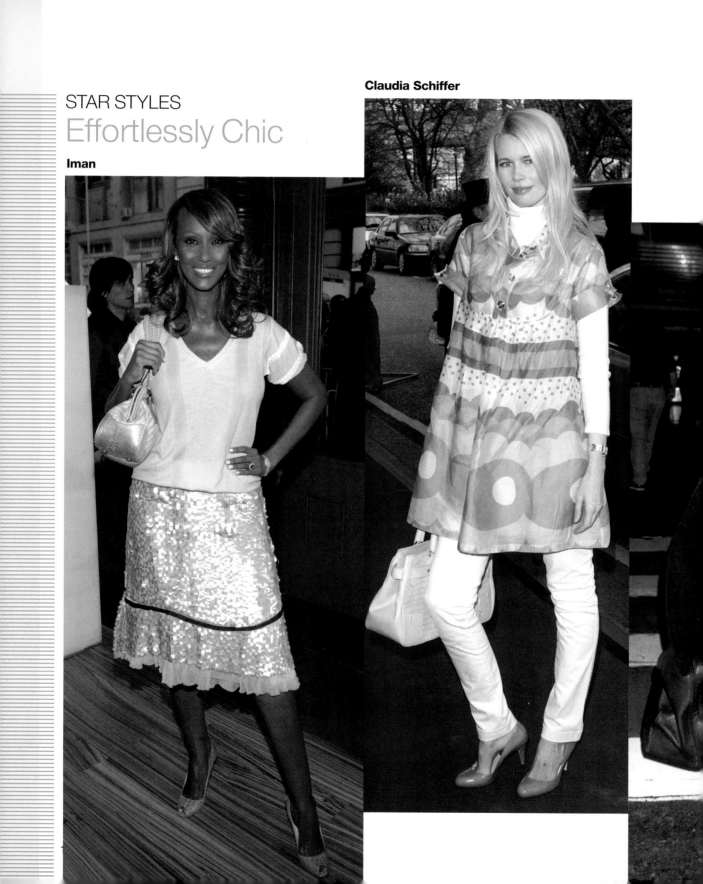

STAR STYLES
Effortlessly Chic

Iman

Claudia Schiffer

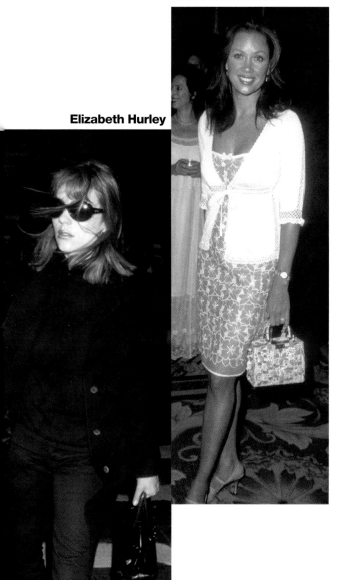

Vanessa Williams

Elizabeth Hurley

GET HELP — FOR FREE!

Are you still having a hard time trying to pull it all together? If yes, take advantage of the best-kept secret in retailing: free fashion advice. All you have to do is book an appointment. If you are shopping for a fresh spring look at, say, Barneys New York, why not enlist the help of one of the best personal shoppers in the biz? Call Sharyn Soleimani's office, tell her what you're shopping for, and she will have a rack of possibilities in your size waiting for you in her spacious private dressing room on the third floor of the Madison Avenue store. She will honestly tell you what looks good and what doesn't and help you with everything you need to complete your perfect look — shoes, stockings, jewelry, bag, and so on. Your total bill will be the same as if you found the pieces yourself. And there's no charge for the water, coffee, or tea!

Almost every major department store in the country has a personal shopping department. Find the person who best understands your style and check in with her or him every season to find out what's hot, what's new, and what's best for you. Or befriend a salesperson at your favorite boutique and designate her as your personal shopper. Have a meeting with her at the beginning of each season about what trends will work for you. Ask her to pull merchandise for you and to give you a call when your size arrives.

Keep Current on Fashion

What's the best way to keep up on trends? Choose your medium: magazines, the Internet, television. Fashion magazines for the over-thirty crowd include *O, More, Vogue, Elle, In Style,* and *W.* Great fashion Web sites to check out include fashionwiredaily.com, fashionweekdaily.com, style.com, and glam.com. For fashion TV, see *Full Frontal Fashion,* the Video Fashion Network, *Fashion File,* and the Style Network. Or, be the ultimate fashion insider and get yourself a subscription to *Women's Wear Daily* or subscribe online.

UNMATCH YOUR WARDROBE

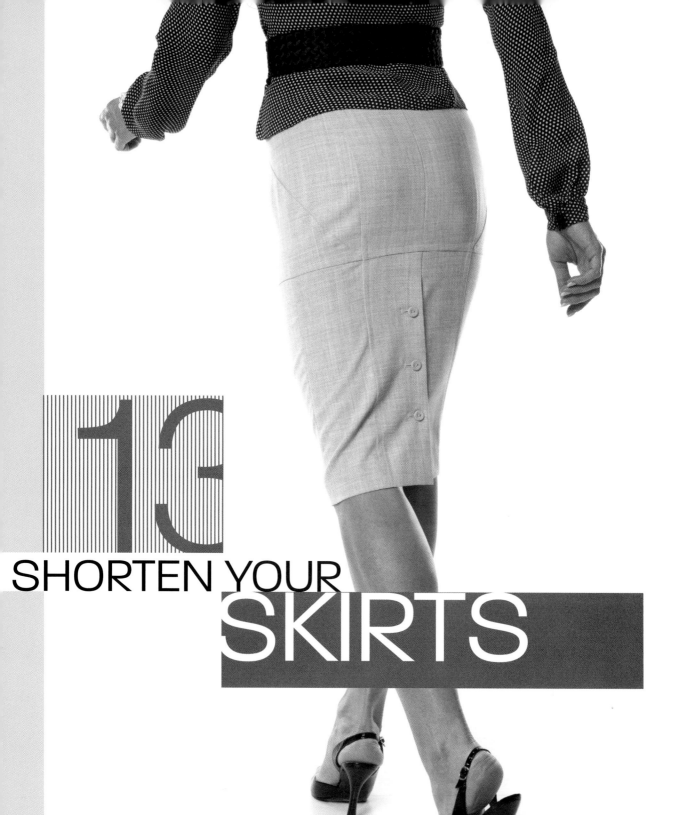

13
SHORTEN YOUR
SKIRTS

NOTHING AGES YOU LIKE...
SKIRTS THAT ARE TOO LONG... TOO SHORT... TOO TIGHT... TOO WIDE... TOO BAGGY... THE WRONG SHAPE... WORN WITH THE WRONG SHOES

When you go to a fashion show and see model after model strutting onto the runway in a crotch-high mini, it's hard to remember that this view of the collection is pure fantasy. This runway routine is designed to play to the cameras and maximize drama, so the clothes you see are much racier than those that end up in the stores. What people outside the fashion business don't realize is that by showtime, the important buyers have already seen the collection and placed their orders for real-world renditions of the designers' skirts, dresses, and blouses. Still, seeing images of sixteen-year-old models who weigh a hundred pounds wearing skirts as short as hot pants is not helpful to a grown woman's psyche. It makes us feel bad and does a number on our collective self-esteem because we know we will *never* look like that. And even if we did have the legs for them, high hems just aren't practical for work, for shopping, for carpooling... Forget it!

In real life, how short can your skirts be? The title of this chapter is "Shorten Your Skirts" because most women are wearing their skirts too long and look dowdy as a result. But too short looks inappropriate, not to mention slutty. Every half inch makes a big difference here.

To get the final word on the perfect skirt length, I've consulted my top style mavens — Sharyn Soleimani at Barneys New York; Susan Sommers, professional fashion coach; and Joseph Ting, the fashion magazines' go-to tailor — and the good news is, we all agree.

YOUR PERFECT SKIRT LENGTH
Okay, here it is: the perfect length that's always in style, that's between trying too hard and looking OL. It's that spot on the back of your knee that curves in slightly, where your upper and lower leg meet. From the front, it's just above the knee. If you like to be a bit more conservative — but still sexy — have your skirts hit the middle of the knee. That way, you are still revealing the entire calf for an elongated look. The reason you don't want to go any longer is that when a skirt hits mid-calf, it visually chops your legs in half, making you look frumpy and your calves huge. "Even if you have a skinny calf, a skirt should never hit you in the middle of the calf," says Sharyn Soleimani, "because that's not the most flattering part of your leg." Once you've tweaked your skirt length, look at the width, too. Sharyn often advises shoppers to narrow their skirts. "Sometimes skirts are too wide," she says. "Narrower is sexier. You can make a skirt short, but if the width is too wide, you look out of it." So while you're at the tailor's (see the section later in this chapter), tweak the width if you need to.

GETTING IT STRAIGHT: YOUR PERFECT SKIRT

If you think I'm going to say let's hear it for the A-line, I'm not. Conventional wisdom says that the A-line, which flares out slightly from the waistband to the hem, is the most universally flattering skirt, and it is. And if you have very

At work, your skirt choice sends a message. You want that message to be that you're someone who "gets it," not "Grandma's in the house!" A simple, well-fitting straight skirt is always appropriate. In creative workplaces, you can get away with a looser, more fashion-y look, such as a tiered and flirty peasant skirt in the summer.

Kiss the Micromini Good-bye!

Last time I saw Tina Turner onstage, she was still wearing microminiskirts. If you've got legs like hers (and also happen to be a performer), then by all means show them off! But for the rest of us, it's time to admit that the micromini is ridiculous. Go ahead and try one on, then look at yourself objectively in the mirror. Bend down, pick up a paper clip, and check out your rear view. I'm sorry, but any skirt that hits four inches or more above the knees is too short for a woman our age. And those "shorts suits" that retailers are pushing? Knees are tricky enough on summer weekends; do you really want to deal with them at the office? You won't look Y&H, but rather as if you're trying too hard to be with it.

thick legs, it can balance you out, like a pair of boot-cut jeans. But the truth is, the A-line is not the hippest skirt. In fact, it is OL. A straight skirt that's fitted to show off your curves looks fresher and more sophisticated. What tailor Joseph Ting does a lot of these days is alter the A-line. "If you want to make it hip, you just taper the ends and make it a straight skirt," he says. "A straight skirt is more chic." And if you still have the bod, a pencil skirt, which is slimmer and more fitted than a straight skirt, is classy yet super-sexy. Another Y&H choice is a fit-and-flared trumpet skirt, which flares out at the bottom and can add curves to slim hips without adding bulk to the legs. The fluidity — that sense of movement in the flounce — can look swingy, which is very Y&H. If you're afraid of feeling lumpy in a straight skirt, the answer is a powerful tummy smoother (see chapter 16), not an OL skirt with a voluminous amount of fabric.

TO STAY OR TO GO? A CHEAT SHEET FOR THE SKIRTS IN YOUR CLOSET

Over the past few seasons, skirts vying for our attention have included the pencil, the mini, the trumpet, the peasant, the balloon, and the dirndl. It's good to know about the new shape of the season, but the older you get, the more you need to edit your skirts and wear only the shapes that look best on you. "You don't want to embrace every trend as fully as you did when you were younger, because you'll look like a walking fashion victim," Susan Sommers advises. "It has to be appropriate for your body type, lifestyle, what you do, and where you do it." Over the years, if you're like me, you've collected a wardrobe of shapes. You already know that all your straight skirts are

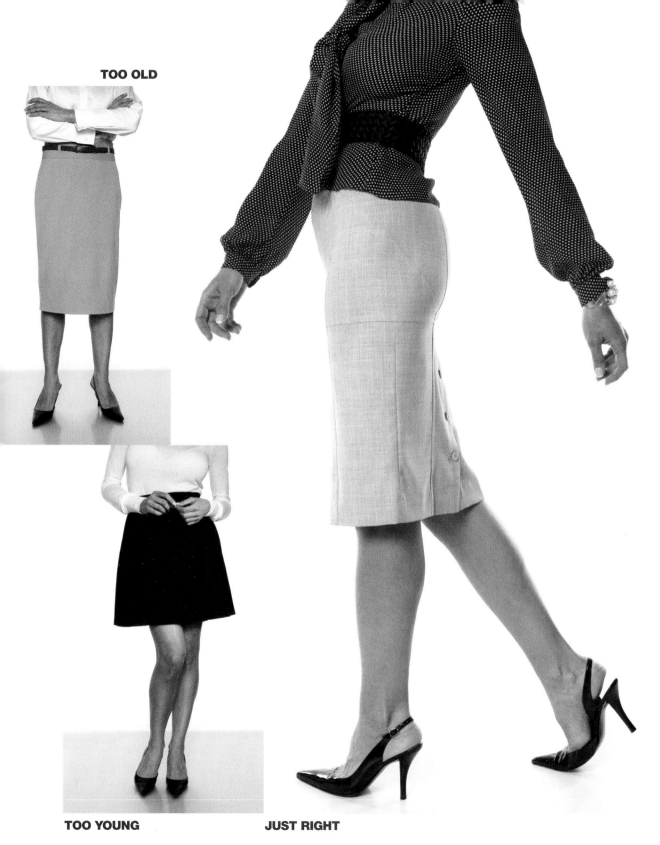

TOO OLD

TOO YOUNG

JUST RIGHT

Your Skirt Is Too Tight If . . .

- It curves in beneath your bottom.
- It "whiskers" in front (which means the fabric is pulling).
- You can see the outline of your pubic bone.
- It's a challenge to walk, sit, or bend.

keepers. Now it's time to take stock of the rest of your skirts.

Balloon skirt: Full and gathered at the waist, then curved toward the knees, this shape can look good on someone with a flat rear end in need of a curve. If you have a curve, you don't need this skirt; you need one that's straighter.

Peasant skirt: This wedding-cake style with multiple tiers and flounces can look costumey on everyone and completely drown a petite. But don't rush to judgment on the entire category. Assess your skirt on its individual merits. A slightly more tailored interpretation, when paired with a small top, can be flirty and fun without making you look like an actual peasant.

Long skirt: Whether you're looking at a casual version or a gown for a black-tie event, long can look OL. It's much more chic to show a little leg.

Pleated skirt: The start-at-the-waist knife pleats popular for grammar school uniforms are a great look — for schoolgirls. Pleats need to be sewn down from the waist to the mid-thigh. Watch the length: short pleated skirts are for cheerleaders.

Denim skirt: Jeans are Y&H; jean skirts are not. They're usually too casual, too stiff, too Daisy Mae, or too cowgirl to be truly flattering.

Full or circle skirt: The voluminous look is tricky on adult women. Leave this very girlish fifties shape to the girls.

Dirndl skirt: "I would say that this is the one no-no skirt for almost everybody our age," says Sommers.

"There's so much puffiness at the waist. It's so hard to wear, but it perennially comes back."

Front-slit skirt: This style is neither flattering nor practical. A small side or back slit will make a straight or pencil skirt easier to walk in (and show a sexy flash of leg). But a front slit is awkward when you sit and reveal inches of thigh better left under wraps. (You don't want to expose your bike shorts!)

THE TAILOR: YOUR NEW BEST FRIEND

An excellent tailor can rescue your mistakes, update an old favorite, or tweak almost anything. "When things fit you perfectly, they look far more expensive than they are," says Susan Sommers. "But expensive things that don't fit you perfectly, don't look good." If you're petite, your tailor has probably been an official member of your fashion posse for years. To get the skinny on what a tailor can do — and whether it's worth the cost — I turned to one of the best in the business, Joseph Ting of Dynasty Tailors in New York City. As I mentioned earlier, he's the one that many fashion magazines call on when they need clothes for a shoot altered by the next day.

When it comes to shoes, the formula is simple: the shorter the skirt, the lower the heel.

The Newer Way to . . .

Pair Tops (and Shoes) with Skirts

When it comes to pulling together the most flattering skirt outfit, think about proportion. The goal is to have an hourglass figure, so you have to show your shape either on the top or the bottom — both pieces cannot be voluminous. A fuller skirt (peasant, balloon, or A-line) requires a more fitted top. "Otherwise, you look wide," says Sharyn Soleimani. "So many people don't get this. When a woman is more mature, she might say, 'I want the top to be more comfortable.' She's not realizing that being comfortable doesn't mean the top has to be voluminous. You can still be comfortable in something that's a bit more fitted." On the flip side, if both pieces are too tight, you'll look trashy. And when it comes to shoes, the formula is simple: the shorter the skirt, the lower the heel.

Always

■ Pair a full, flirty summer skirt with a fitted T-shirt or tank top.

■ Try a trim blouse under a slim V-neck sweater with a skirt that's fitted and flouncy, not clingy. If the sweater is a little shorter than the blouse, better yet. It's a more modern, very Y&H look.

■ Elongate legs with high-heeled boots and matching tights. A snug pair of knee-high boots works like magic to slim calves and give legs a great long look.

■ Wear some kind of heel with knee-length skirts. Even with long, thin legs, flats can look dowdy.

Never

■ Pair bulky with bulky (such as a full skirt with a big sweater).

■ Wear too tight with too tight. A super-slim pencil skirt will look trashy with a skintight bustier or tube top, but classy with a tailored shirt or feminine blouse.

■ Slip on stilettos with a super-short skirt. It's a recipe for disaster — and call girls.

■ Assume that blouses and tops need to be tucked in. Out looks fresher.

Y&H Skirts . . . Hitting the Right Length

Sela Ward   **Vanessa Williams**   **Diane Sawyer**

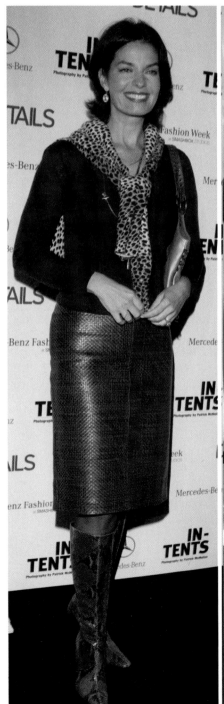
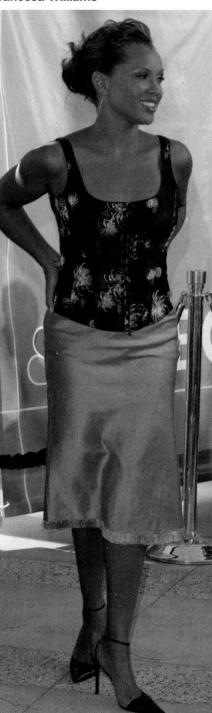
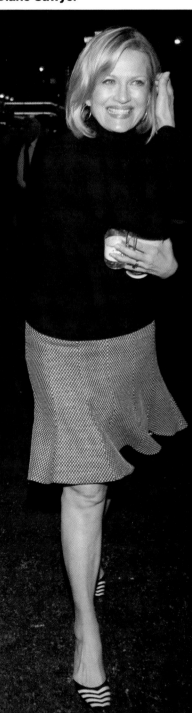

What the Tailor Can Do

■ Shorten your skirts. Any that fall below your knees should get hiked up.

■ Straighten your skirts. Joseph takes dowdy A-lines and tailors them into Y&H straight skirts. This simple alteration tapers the ends to create a classic line that will never go out of style. (At Dynasty, this costs $49.)

■ Lift your waistline. If you have a skirt that rests too low on your hips, have a tailor cinch it in at the waist so that it sits just under your belly button and doesn't feel as if it's slipping off. (Also about $49 at Dynasty.)

■ Shorten a jacket. A long suit jacket that falls at mid-thigh is so OL — and so nineties. Joseph often crops jackets that don't have pockets in the way.

■ Nip in a jacket at the waist. A tighter fit makes for a tinier waist, so a couple of darts in the back may salvage a jacket you love.

■ Replace shoulder pads. You know that those old linebacker-style shoulder pads have to go. A tailor can swap them out for smaller, softer, more natural-looking versions.

What Isn't Worth Salvaging

Sometimes you just have to be strong and send your clothes off into the universe to find another woman who will enjoy them as you once did. (Check out bottomlesscloset.org.) Alterations on the following items just aren't worth the cost.

■ Inexpensive items. Joseph recommends saving the major overhauls for designer pieces. Spending $100 to fix a skirt that cost less than that probably isn't a wise investment.

■ Long, oversized jackets with pockets or belts. They can't be shortened, so good-bye to the eighties and nineties.

■ Trendy shapes or colors. If something's out of style, it's not worth the investment. It's better to tailor classics in classic colors — black, brown, beige, gray, navy — that have staying power.

■ Anything you don't really love. Don't compound the mistake. If it's too late to return it, cut your losses, donate it to charity, and at least get a tax break.

SIZE DOESN'T MATTER — BUT FIT DOES!

When I was at *Shop Etc.* magazine, we sent a size 8 fit model into eleven stores and had her try on various designer trousers to see which sizes fit. Our model was trying on pants, but the results of our survey translate to skirts as well. Use these guidelines the next time you head to the dressing room. *

Store	Size That Fit	Shopping Rule
Ann Taylor	6	Cut big. Drop down a size.
Banana Republic	4	Cut really big. Drop down two sizes.
Club Monaco	6	Cut big. Drop down a size.
Donna Karan	6	Cut big. Drop down a size.
Gap	6	Cut big. Drop down a size.
Giorgio Armani	6	Cut big. Drop down a size.
Gucci	8	Perfect fit!
H&M	10	Cut small. Go up a size.
J. Crew	6	Cut big. Drop down a size.
L. L. Bean	8	Perfect fit!
Ralph Lauren	8	Perfect fit!

*Originally appeared in *Shop Etc.*, a publication of Hearst Communications, Inc.

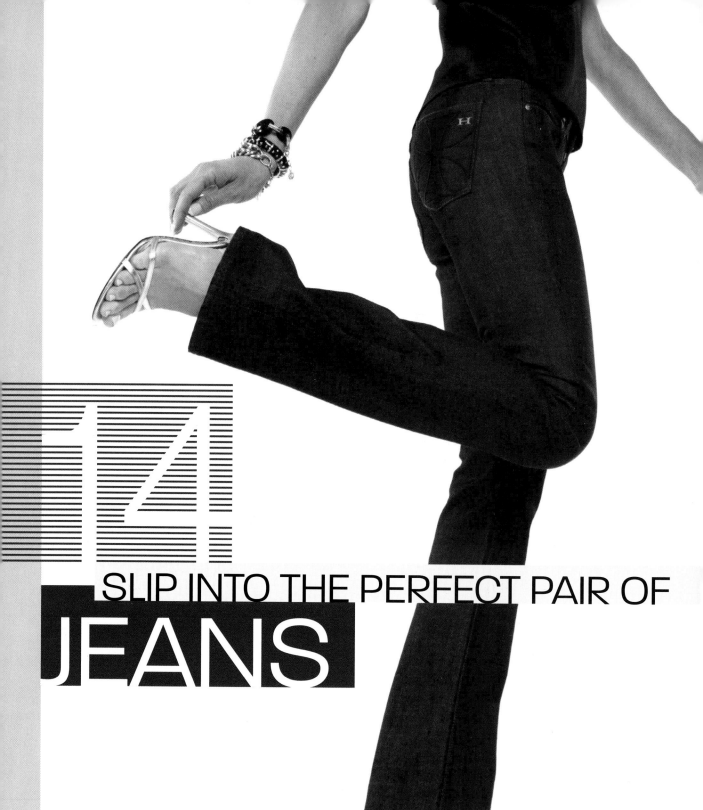

14.
SLIP INTO THE PERFECT PAIR OF
JEANS

NOTHING AGES YOU LIKE...
ELASTIC WAISTBANDS... MOMMY JEANS... HIGH-RISE JEANS... FADED JEANS... BAGGY JEANS... EMBELLISHED JEANS... FLASHING YOUR THONG AND BUTT CLEAVAGE... EXPOSING YOUR LOVE HANDLES... JEANS THAT ARE TOO TIGHT... YOUR DAUGHTER'S JEANS

You say you don't wear jeans? Then you are missing out on the one item of clothing that has replaced the little black dress as the must-have staple of every Y&H wardrobe. I'm a total convert now — with five dark denim pairs and one white pair currently hanging in my closet. But as recently as 2001, I wouldn't be caught dead in jeans. I did a segment on jeans for the *Today* show, but I wasn't even wearing them myself. If Katie Couric had called me on it, I was prepared to say, "You know I'd do anything for *Today* viewers — except wear jeans or a bathing suit on the air!"

Flash forward to July 2003. I was taping a segment for the TBS show *Movie & a Makeover* about Barneys New York Denim Bar. Surrounded by the latest styles from all the top labels, I bought my first pair of jeans since college. I've since appeared on the *Today* show in jeans — in jeans segments and even when the segments aren't about jeans. Why? I look better in my jeans than in any other piece of clothing in my closet.

If you can't make the same statement, it's because you haven't found the right pair of jeans. But once you do, you won't know how you ever lived without them. You really need to have several pairs — ideally three or four — for dressing up, shopping on a Saturday, hanging around the house, and maybe even for work (depending on your job). No matter what your age, nothing says Y&H faster than a perfect pair of jeans. Jeans are forever cool. Of course, the right pair is crucial. The wrong pair will simply make you look OL — or, worse, as if you're trying too hard to look young.

The reason that so many women haven't put on a pair of jeans since their embroidered ones in college is that for a long time, jeans really weren't that flattering. They made our butts look big and our thighs look thick. Jeans made us look dumpy. But that has completely changed over the past several years. According to Cotton Incorporated, women today own an average of eight pairs of jeans, and there are currently more than three hundred labels vying for your rear end. Many of those manufacturers have wised up and realized that it's not only teens and twentysomethings who are buying jeans. Shoppers ages 35 to 44 purchase more jeans than any other age group, and those 55 to 65 are the fastest-growing group of denim buyers. Why? Because of the new styles, more flattering fits, and sophisticated details, zillions of jeans now work like a dream to make us look Y&H.

GREAT FIT: THE PRICE OF PERFECTION

With the dizzying array of brands and styles out there, finding the perfect pair of jeans can seem even more overwhelming than buying a swimsuit. But what separates a great pair that'll take ten years off from one that's OL can be summed up in one word: fit. And fit is a big part of what you're paying for when you look at brands with price tags in the triple digits. According to Cotton Incorporated, 85 percent of jeans shoppers say that fit is their number one concern, and most of us say that we'd actually pay up to 28 percent more for jeans with the right fit.

It's a jeans truism that the younger you are and the better body you have, the more you can get away with an inexpensive pair of jeans. In 2004, when I did a *Today* segment on great-fitting jeans with Natalie Morales, the only person who looked amazing in the $19 pair was my twenty-year-old intern. It's not that I *want* to pay more for a designer label; it's just that pricier jeans are better engineered and every detail is thought through to flatter the body perfectly.

Prices keep inching up, but most designer jeans cost somewhere between $150 and $250. Cotton Incorporated says that only 4 percent of jeans fall into the premium category (which they define as costing more than $60!). To me, the moral of that story is, most people go for low-price jeans, and some look like hell in them. Just because you find a pair of jeans that fits over your body doesn't mean that they're flattering. If the fabric doesn't bend, the shape doesn't suit your curves, or the legs make your thighs look huge, they are not the right jeans for you. But if you can buy a pair for $20 that makes you look amazing and gives you a great butt, bravo!

Cool jeans are an investment. I probably get more wear out of my jeans than out of anything else I own. I'm still wearing the pair I bought in 2003. If you take good care of them (see the section on caring for denim), they'll last for years.

Don't assume that you can bring just one pair of jeans into the dressing room and find The One. More likely, you'll pull on and off a dozen or so pairs, so shop when you have the time and the patience to try and try and try. To make the task a little less overwhelming, find a store that not only carries several brands but has sales staff who really know their stuff. You want an expert who can quickly size you up and hand you several pairs to get the process started. Some department stores are known for their jeans selection, such as Barneys New York's legendary Denim Bar, where the "bartender" in residence will do just that. Smaller specialty stores that have popped up in cities across the country carry the hottest names and can quickly help you find the pair that looks best on your butt.

Of course, it doesn't pay to get too attached to any one label. Jeans brands have become like handbags: there's an "it" name every season. And even though they could be the coolest jeans on the planet, if they don't flatter your butt, they're not Y&H. Pay attention to how good your rear end looks, not whose label is on it.

IT'S ALL IN THE DETAILS

"There is nothing that is going to age you faster than the wrong-fitting jeans," says Susan Sommers, fashion coach. The stars need to align on several elements to create a jeans look that is unmistakably Y&H. The right pair of jeans can take off not only ten years but ten pounds as well. Here are the details every smart shopper needs to know.

The right rise: One of the key elements in how a pair of jeans fit is the "rise" — the distance from the crotch seam to the top of the waistband. There are two ways to go wrong here. At one extreme,

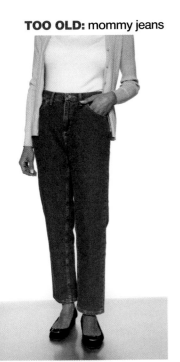

TOO OLD: mommy jeans

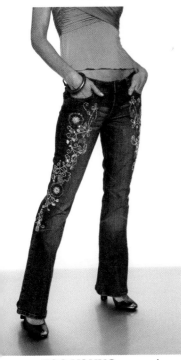

TOO YOUNG: super-low and overembellished

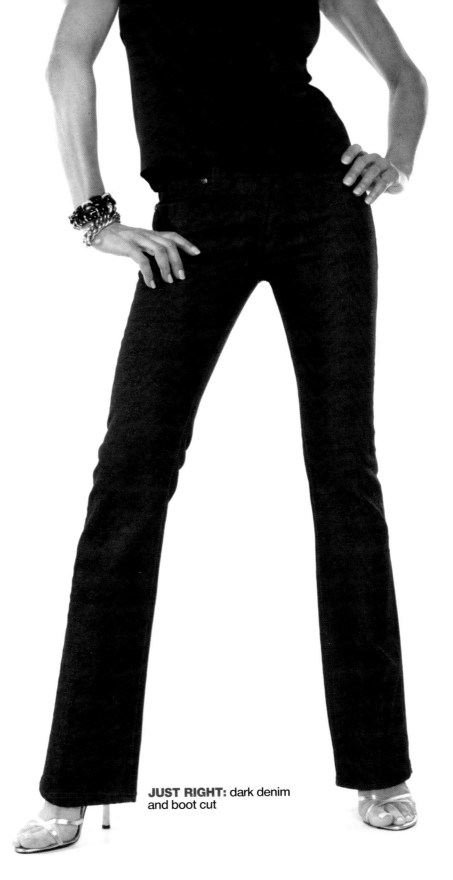

JUST RIGHT: dark denim and boot cut

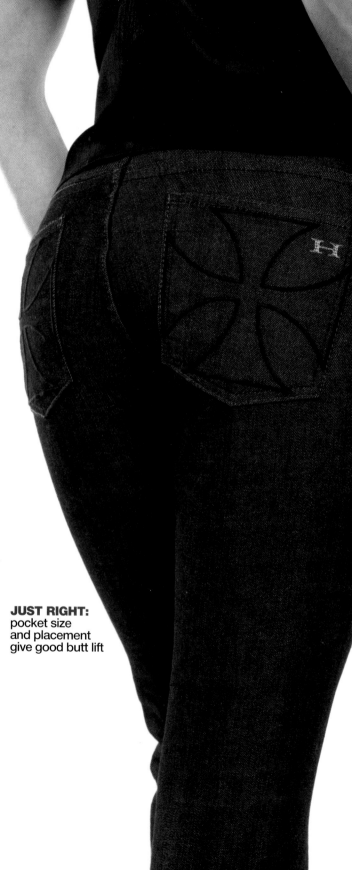

jeans that ride really low on the hips are for teenagers. (Plus, a low rise can expose love handles you never even realized you had!) At the other extreme, jeans that come all the way up to your waist scream OL. These are the quintessential "mommy jeans," and there is absolutely nothing sexy about them. The high rise makes hips look hippier, tummy pouffier, and butt and thighs fuller than they need to.

What you want is a mid–low-rise. If you have to bring a tape measure with you when you shop, do it. You're looking for an eight- to nine-inch rise — still well below the belly button, but not too low. As Sharyn Soleimani puts it, "Bending over and having your underwear show . . . What's flattering about that at *any* age? Nothing!"

Some designers have come up with a clever, have-it-both-ways solution: jeans that ride low in front but significantly higher in back. One example is Stella jeans from Chip & Pepper. (See the jeans cheat sheet later in this chapter.)

The right color: The wash (the color finish of the fabric) is your next consideration when faced with a sea of jeans in varying shades of indigo. There are only two worth wearing — true blue and dark wash. And the simpler the better: no holes or tears, no glittery embellishments, no embroidery. Faded washes don't do your figure any favors, nor do "whiskers" — those wispy little lines that radiate out from your crotch and call unwanted attention to your hips.

The right shape: There's a reason boot-cut jeans are still most women's favorite: they do our hips a huge favor. Thanks to the slight flare at the bottom, this is the best style for balancing out your body. The right boot-cut jeans have a nineteen-inch leg opening. For the office, an even better option is a pair of trouser jeans. They're cut more like a pair of nice pants than a pair of jeans, with a wider leg, a flat front, and a wider waistband. Look for a pair without belt loops for an even sleeker silhouette.

JUST RIGHT:
pocket size
and placement
give good butt lift

Then there's the skinny jean. It has a straight, tight silhouette and a meager twelve-inch leg opening. Unless your body is equally straight and skinny, this style will look too tight, too young, and not very flattering. If you want the feeling of this trendy shape, try a straight-leg jean. The slim silhouette will make your legs look long and lean. The straight-leg style is like the skinny, just not quite so legging-like.

The right fabric: Jeans with just a touch of stretch will hug your curves and move with your body without pulling or tugging. But they shouldn't be so stretchy that they could be mistaken for leggings. The ideal proportion is 2 or 3 percent Lycra spandex and 97 or 98 percent cotton — just enough stretch to make you comfortable, but not enough that anyone but you will know. If the percentage of stretch is higher than 3 percent, the jeans will be too tight (the dreaded "sausage" feeling). Jeans with no stretch aren't as comfortable, especially when you're sitting down. They're also more likely to gap at the waist or sag after a few hours.

The right pockets: It may not seem that complicated to put together a pair of jeans, but their design has become a science all its own. Every seam, stitch, and grommet is placed purposefully to maximize the jeans' figure-flattering potential. Pocket size, shape, and placement separate the perfect pair from the stack of rejects you leave in the dressing room. Be on the lookout for pockets that are too small (especially if you worry that your butt is too big). Little pockets leave too much surface area uncovered, and that emphasizes a

Nip and Tuck

It's trendy at the moment to tuck jeans inside your boots. Obviously, the skinnier the jeans, the easier this is to pull off. But this trick from fashion stylist Genevieve Yraola works like a charm, even with boot-cut jeans. Fold over your jeans to make them tight around your ankle, then slip a wide rubber band around them. This will hold the jeans snug so you can pull on your boots without the fabric bunching up around your legs.

generous tush. You want pockets that occupy the entire expanse from the bottom of the rise to the edge of your butt. Larger pockets, those set lower on the seat, and those angled slightly will give your rear a visual lift. The style of the stitching also has the power to improve your bottom line. Paper Denim & Cloth's Mod jeans have stitching that curves around just the outer edges of the pockets to draw eyes in and create the optical illusion of slimmer hips.

JEANS' BEST FRIENDS

Now that you've got the perfect pair, you need the right accoutrements to complete the look.

The right shoes: Not all jeans look good with all shoes. Please don't wear gym sneakers with jeans. Let the width of the leg opening determine the perfect shoe pairing. Fashion stylist Genevieve Yraola, who styled the models in this book, came up with this new rule: the narrower the cut, the more delicate your shoes need to be. So if you choose skinny jeans, wear them with a slim kitten heel or sleek stiletto. Straight-leg jeans look best with a delicate pump (a d'Orsay style, with cutout sides, shows off a little skin and is a sexy complement to long, leggy jeans) or a pointy-toe boot. As the leg gets wider, your shoes should get a little sturdier. Boot-cut jeans pair up nicely with a slightly thicker-heeled boot or Mary Janes, and wide-leg trouser jeans look chic and professional paired with platform pumps or a chunky-heeled boot.

The right undies: With jeans, the undies issue isn't so much VPL (visible panty line) as it is VTE (visible thong exposure). Even if you avoid low low-rise jeans, you run the risk of flashing your thong — or, worse, your butt cleavage — every time you sit down. Look for thongs that have a slight V dip in the rear to ensure that they stay out of sight (see Brilliant Buys in chapter 16).

YOUR SHOPPING SURVIVAL GUIDE: TIPS TO TAKE TO THE DRESSING ROOM

■ **Focus.** If you want dark blue jeans, don't get sidetracked trying on a stack of jeans in a lighter wash.

■ **To save time** going back and forth from the dressing room to the racks, bring two sizes — the one you think you are, plus one size up or down — of each style to the dressing room.

■ **Wear the boots** or shoes that you plan to wear with the jeans. Put the shoes on and tuck the hem of the jeans under to the right length to get a true sense of how they'll look.

■ **Sit down** in the jeans. They should feel snug, but if they're cutting off your circulation, they are either too small or the wrong cut for your body. Also check for a gap in the back of the waistband. A tailor can fix a small gap, but if there's more than an inch to spare, try another pair.

■ **Squat** and check out your rear view in a mirror. If the super-low thong you're wearing is exposed, the rise is too low.

■ **Look at the back pockets** in a three-way mirror. This is your moment of truth. If your butt doesn't look fantastic, keep trying!

Your Size Guide

Sizing is not consistent from brand to brand, and pairs from pricier lines will run smaller than brands such as Gap and Lee. Here's a guide to get you started.

Waist (inches)	Size Equivalent
24	0
25	0–2
26	2
27	4
28	6
29	8
30	8–10
31	10–12
32	12
33	12–14
34	14

Please don't wear gym sneakers with jeans. Let the width of the leg opening determine the perfect shoe pairing.

HIGH, MEDIUM, AND LOW MAINTENANCE . . . SHOPPING FOR JEANS

You need to own at least two pairs that are dark denim, boot-cut, mid–low-rise. Here are three ways to get the look.

HIGH: You'll spare no expense when it comes to finding flattering jeans, and you buy several pairs every season to stay up-to-date with the latest labels and silhouettes. You should have a whole wardrobe of jeans to suit different moods and occasions — trousers for work; jeans hemmed for flats, heels, and in between; a dressy pair in black velvet for a night on the town; a white pair for summer. And why not go all the way and get a pair custom-made just for you? At an Earnest Cut & Sew shop in New York City's meatpacking district, you can pick your fabric, fit, finish, and pocket details and have a pair made right on the premises.

MEDIUM: You're willing to pay the price (and realize that price will be $150 or more) for jeans that will make you look Y&H. Make sure you have one pair hemmed for flats and one for dressier heels. Put yourself in the hands of the denim experts at a store that is known for its vast selection and personal assistance. Do-it-yourselfers can check out dozens of options at zafu.com — a Web site that offers a detailed quiz about your preferences, then links you to your best brands.

LOW: Jeans for less than $50 are available from the Gap, Lee, and Levi's. Mass retailers such as Target carry Levi Strauss Signature jeans (about $20).

STAR STYLES
Big Names in Jeans

Sheryl Crow

Diane Keaton

Claudia Schiffer

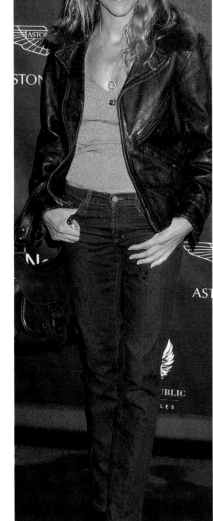

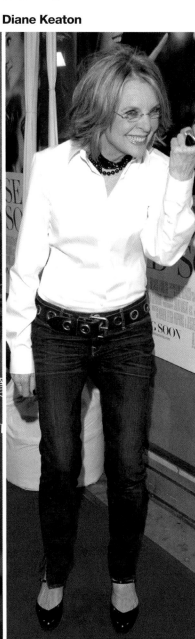

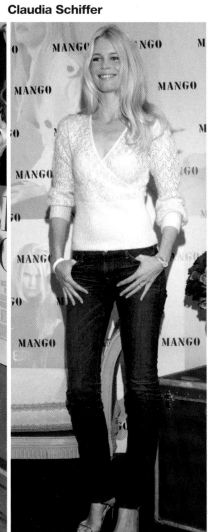

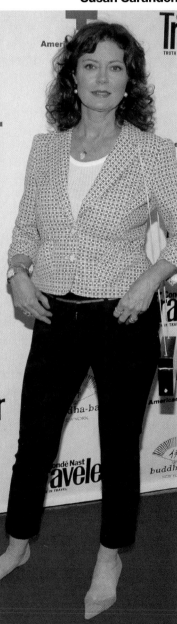

Teri Hatcher   **Susan Sarandon**

FINE-TUNE YOUR FIT

Don't forget about the tailor when you're shopping for jeans. Unless you're supermodel tall, you will need to have your jeans hemmed. Wearing a pair that's dragging on the floor or rolled into cuffs is not Y&H — it's too young and messy. You want your jeans to look as chic and sophisticated as a beautiful pair of trousers.

Wash your jeans before you have them hemmed. Most manufacturers claim that the fabrics are preshrunk, but they still shrink slightly in length at first. Then take them to the tailor along with the shoes you plan to wear with them. Skinny or straight-leg jeans can be hemmed slightly long to wear with heels and will scrunch up nicely when you wear flats. But boot-cut jeans need to be hemmed to the exact length for the heels you plan to wear with them. That's why you should consider buying two pairs — even if they're the exact same jeans: one that's hemmed for flats, the other for heels.

The right length hits one-eighth to one-quarter inch from the ground. Don't go too short, warns Susan Sommers. "One or two inches can be the difference between looking like you're wearing mommy jeans or cool jeans," she says. And be sure to ask the tailor to use the original hem. That means that the tailor cuts off the original hem, shortens the jeans, and then invisibly reattaches the hem. A new hem will look too "perfect" — okay for trousers, but too OL for a hip pair of jeans. Genevieve Yraola suggests Radcliffe jeans, which offer a solution for a variety of shoe heights. They're made with hidden cuff links that can lengthen or hike up the hem.

CARING FOR YOUR DENIM INVESTMENT

Dry-clean or machine-wash? Tumble or hang dry? Your choice will dictate how your jeans look, as well as how long they last. There's no doubt that dry-cleaning will keep the color from fading, but that pressed look will make your jeans a little too fussy

The right length hits one-eighth to one-quarter inch from the ground.

and OL. If you dry-clean anything, make it your dressier, trouser-style jeans that you wear to work.

Always turn your jeans inside out before washing to preserve the color, and wash them in cold water on the gentle cycle. Jeans with stretch should never go in the dryer (the heat will break down the elastic fibers). If you have an all-cotton pair that you need to shrink back into shape, toss them in the dryer on low. Otherwise, hang your jeans to dry.

The Newer Way to . . .
Wear Jeans

Please Do
■ **Buy the pair that makes your butt look its best,** regardless of whether or not it's the label du jour.
■ **Choose the smaller size if you're on the fence.** Jeans will always stretch out a bit, so if you buy the pair that's a little too large, they'll end up looking too baggy and OL.
■ **Wear boot-cut or straight-leg jeans.** Anything else will give you an unbalanced silhouette and make your hips and rear look bigger.
■ **Choose the simplest, least embellished styles you can find.** Ones with lots of glitz are too young-looking.

Please Don't
■ **Wear baggy jeans** or jeans with a rolled-up cuff.
■ **Wear jeans with strange — and unflattering — distress patterns** on the thighs or butt.
■ **Wear jeans with "dirty" washes.** The name says it all. Grungy jeans are a definite no-no.
■ **Wear two pieces of denim clothing at once.** Choose either pants or a jacket, not both.
■ **Assume that all butt-booster jeans will be flattering.** Some simply flatten you out rather than give a sexy shape.

Your Jeans Cheat Sheet: A Guide to Miracle Workers in Denim

New styles and labels are born every season. Following is a very subjective list of a few favorites bound to flatter. Consider these the brands that have earned the "How Not to Look Old" seal of approval.

AG Jeans: Oprah loves them, too. There's a cut for every body, including a universally flattering slight boot-cut with stretch and pockets that sit lower on the rear (which gives the butt a lift).

Chip & Pepper: The Stella jeans, with a 7½-inch rise in the front and an 11½-inch rise in the back, allow low-rise lovers to stay covered.

Citizens of Humanity: The designer, Jean Paul Duhomme, was one of the creators of 7 for All Mankind. His own line is equally chic and stays fashionable season after season. Look for dark indigo rinses and office-appropriate trouser styles.

Habitual: The classic boyfriend jeans are known for their great fit and clever graduated waistband that ensures complete rear coverage.

James Cured by Seun: These jeans are perfect for women like us for two reasons: (1) the styles (even the straight-leg versions) take curves into account and flatter them with perfect pocket placement, and (2) they are utterly unembellished. Even the seams are devoid of visible topstitching, so the result is a lean, clean line.

Joe's Jeans: The contoured fit through the hips and butt makes these jeans perfect for those who need a little extra room in the rear. Some styles rise higher in the back for better coverage.

Paige Premium Denim: Paige Adams Geller was a fit model for many of the top denim lines, and she's taken all she learned from those designers and created her own amazing brand of premium jeans. Her styles are classic, chic, and comfortable, with an emphasis on fit over trendiness.

Paper Denim & Cloth: This brand is famous for its flattering fit that still provides full coverage in the rear. All styles feature clever pocket stitching that visually slims the hips.

Salt Jeans: "A lot of women who are older cannot stand jeans that are cut low on the waist," says Sharyn Soleimani. "When Salt Jeans came out, I said, 'Finally, someone is cutting jeans a little higher on the waist.' "

7 for All Mankind: These have been around since the beginning of the jeans revolution and are still popular among celebrities. Known for their slim fit through the thigh and clean lines.

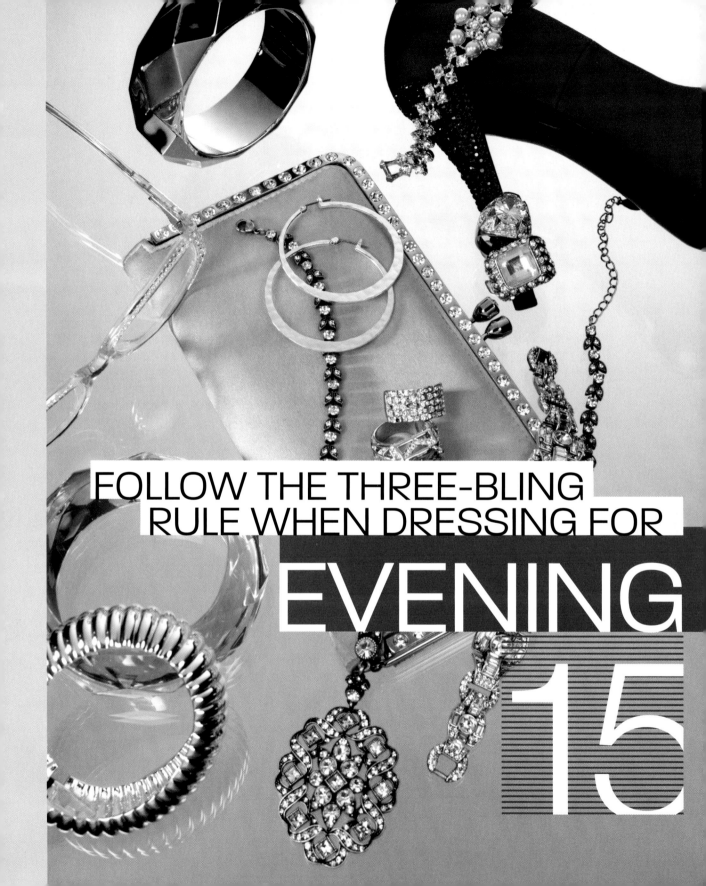

FOLLOW THE THREE-BLING
RULE WHEN DRESSING FOR

EVENING

15

NOTHING AGES YOU LIKE ...
OVERBLING ... EXPOSING TOO MUCH SKIN ... SHOWING EXCESSIVE CLEAVAGE ... BEARLIKE MINK COATS ... OUTDATED JEWELRY ... OVER-SIZED EARRINGS ... TIGHTLY WOUND HAIR ... SPARKLY MAKEUP ... FRAGRANCE OVERLOAD

Too many of us make the mistake of piling on every shiny, glitzy, fancy thing we own when we get dressed up for a big evening. The result? Serious overbling! It's not Y&H to be blinging on all burners: Necklace! Earrings! Shoes! Bag! But it's *so* easy to overdo it. This chapter is about how not to go into panic mode when you see the words "black tie."

I, too, have rushed around like a lunatic at the last minute, trying on different shoes, bracelets, earrings, necklaces — while simultaneously smoothing bronzer on my legs and trying to stuff the contents of my everyday handbag into a teeny evening clutch and forcing it to close. The anxiety! Over the years, getting ready for events such as the Oscars, Emmys, Grammys, and Tonys, I've learned that whatever time you allot to prepping, it will *never* be enough.

One secret to looking great is to take care of yourself as much as possible ahead of time. Preparedness is key. I'm not suggesting that you devote weeks to the project of getting ready for a single night out, but some simple strategies, such as having a "black-tie prop kit" readily available in your closet (see the section later in this chapter), will go a long way toward ensuring a gorgeous result. And it may even make you happy to see the words "black tie" on an invitation.

WHERE IT ALL BEGINS: ONE GREAT DRESS

Most of us head out shopping for a special-occasion dress when the pressure is on, just days before the event. It's a better idea to shop for an evening dress when there is no imminent invitation. That's when you're most likely to stumble on the dress of your dreams or find a fabulous dress on sale. So whenever you're shopping — especially during postholiday sales — always have an eye out for a great evening dress in a classic shape, style, and color. Because wouldn't it be great to have it hanging in your closet — tailored and ready to wear — when the invite arrives? And when someone asks you that dreaded question, "What are you going to wear?" you already know.

What's the best style for your evening dress? Before you decide whether to go strapless, short, long, sleeveless, backless, or plunging neckline, decide what part of your body you want to show off. Looking Y&H and sexy at a formal affair means revealing some skin — whether it's your legs, back, shoulders, arms, or cleavage. Remember that a little skin goes a long way, so choose just one area to bare. You want to show off your assets, but overexposure can translate as "desperate," which isn't sexy at any age.

How do you decide what to bare? Well, what's best about you? The old rules dictating that women over a certain age shouldn't go strapless or show cleavage (or any other hard-and-fast rules) no longer apply, since women now work out like crazy and may be in the best shape of their lives. So if you have a firm neck, wear strapless. If you have clear, smooth skin on your chest, show some décolletage. If your arms have great muscle tone, go sleeveless. You know your body well enough to do an honest assessment. Also, trust your gut. You don't have to poll your husband or your mother or your sister or your friends. If you have to ask the question "Am I showing too much?" the answer is yes; otherwise you wouldn't be asking! Keep looking until you find a dress that makes you look fabulous and feel completely confident.

Ban Excessive Boobage

Maybe you've still got great breasts — or just had a lift you want to show off — but when it comes to cleavage, a little goes a long way. When a woman reveals too much, it makes everyone around her nervous, just waiting for a wardrobe malfunction. If you really want to be the one everyone's talking about the day after the party, put it all out there on display. Otherwise, a little mystery is much classier than letting it all hang out.

DRESS FOR SUCCESS STYLES

■ **Strapless:** This style will show off a lot of skin from the chest up, so don't go there unless your neckline and décolletage look beautiful. If your shoulders and upper chest are in good shape, strapless is a classic shape that never goes out of style. If you're big-busted, this might not be your best dress, as the fact that it's cut straight across the chest can make you look top-heavy.

■ **V-neck:** It can highlight great cleavage and create the appearance of an elongated neck. Provided you don't plunge too low, a V-neck can give the illusion of showing more than it actually does.

■ **Three-quarter sleeves:** An excellent choice for anyone with arms that are less than buff. It will provide the perfect camouflage without making you look too covered up.

■ **Sleeveless:** For those who regularly work out and have the strong, toned arms to show for it, sleeveless is always sexy. If you're wearing sleeveless but don't love your arms, look for a little shrug to cover up.

■ **Low back:** Back "cleavage" can be even sexier than the traditional plunging neckline. You don't have to dip as low as some of the stars on the red carpet, but a dress that drapes to the mid-back can look amazing.

■ **Slit skirt:** One that shows a more subtle flash of leg is much sexier than a slit up to there, while still looking classy.

■ **Long vs. short:** For all but the most ultra-formal affairs, any length from knee to shoe is acceptable these days for a black-tie event. Choose the length depending on whether you want to show off shapely legs or hide less-than-perfect ones. But too long can look dowdy.

■ **Separates:** It may seem tempting to buy a dressy skirt or pants that you can mix with different tops, but a dress is going to make more of a "wow!" statement. Plus, it's easier. So many times, those separate pieces don't really work together, and you end up panicking at the last second and trying to shop for another top. Also, evening suits (which can look uptight) and tuxedos (which look better on tall women) are not as Y&H as a sexy dress.

WHY YOU NEED AN LBD

The "little black dress" has been fashion code for a chic classic for so many years now that you might think the whole idea was too clichéd to deserve real estate in your closet. But as Isaac Mizrahi says, "There's nothing more true than a cliché. A little black dress for evening is still the most charming, fabulous thing ever."

You really do need at least one perfect black dress. It's your evening basic — a blank canvas that you can accessorize up and down a zillion different ways and wear over and over and over again. Make sure to buy one in all-season fabric for the most versatility (you can't wear black velvet to a party in July) and in a style that flatters your figure. It will serve as the perfect backdrop to all those drop-dead accessories that are too glitzy for more embellished dresses — like a bold, chunky necklace; sexy, jeweled sandals; or a lacy or patterned wrap.

Everyday Diamonds

It's very OL to think of your "good" jewelry as something that should be kept in a vault and dragged out only on special occasions. It's a habit that comes from the same era as using the "good" china just for holidays and sitting in the living room only when company comes over. It's much more Y&H to wear your jewelry every day. Diamonds with jeans, for instance, looks modern. Besides, what are you saving this stuff for? At the pace it goes in and out of style, you should bring it out and enjoy it while you can!

A great dress that you will wear on several occasions is an investment, so expect to pay a bit more. Luckily, more and more high-end designers are coming out with lower-priced lines, so a well-made dress can still be affordable. Avoid junior lines or any labels made more for the prom set — they won't have the quality you need in the details or the support in the structure of the dress.

And if you don't want to wear black — or you're looking for options to expand your wardrobe of dresses — try a rich jewel tone (burgundy, emerald green, or sapphire). A lot of celebrities wear white, nude, or blush on the red carpet. It's flashy but very hard to wear, can make you look five pounds heavier, and shows every bulge.

THE FUN PART: JEWELRY

Once you've decided on the dress, it's time to start thinking about what jewelry you want to wear with it. Now this is where you might need to rein in your accessorizing impulses. The idea isn't to grab every piece of "good" jewelry in your possession and pile it on. Sharyn Soleimani from Barneys New York says it makes you look insecure, as if "this is the last time you are ever going to see these people, so you want to make sure that they know everything you own!"

Diamonds are forever; jewelry is not. Nothing ages you faster than wearing pieces that were in a decade or two ago. Jewelry designer R. J. Graziano, whose gems appear in all the fashion magazines and jewelry departments (Bloomingdale's, Nordstrom, and Saks), makes this comparison: "You can tell the moment you walk into someone's home if the person is eighty years old or thirty years old. That's [also] how it is with jewelry." His advice is to put those pricey but passé pieces away in the drawer for now. Most likely they will come back in style, but wearing a delicate tennis bracelet when big cuffs rule will make you look like a relic.

When selecting your jewels, R.J.'s advice is to "ask yourself, 'Would a thirty-year-old woman wear this, or does it look like a rich old lady?' Wearing the jewelry of the moment can take twenty years off of you."

■ **Necklace:** A naked neck can be dramatic and elegant, but if you're going to wear a necklace, wear one that makes a statement. Much better a bold, spectacular fake than a teeny, tiny diamond solitaire that gets lost on your neck. The shape and style of the necklace are also important, and they have to complement the neckline of the dress. A necklace that ends in a V can be very

Rx for Earlobe Droop

Add earlobes to the list of things that start to sag at some point. "Aging alone makes the earlobe lengthen," says Dr. Allan Wulc, who offers patients in his Warrington, PA, dermatology practice their leftover Restylane (a hyaluronic acid filler used to plump up wrinkles; see chapter 8) as a way to fix the earring hole's "angle of the dangle." Wearing lots of heavy chandelier earrings contributes to the droop. Ditto sleeping or talking on the phone with earrings on. I actually had Dr. Wulc inject a small amount of Restylane into my earlobes, and ten minutes later, the diamond studs once headed south were shining straight-on. It doesn't hurt, and Dr. Wulc predicts that the results can last up to two years. A syringe of Restylane is expensive ($600 in Dr. Wulc's practice), which is why this "good to the last drop" idea is genius. "The response has been overwhelming. A lot of women get really excited about this," he told me. Who knew?

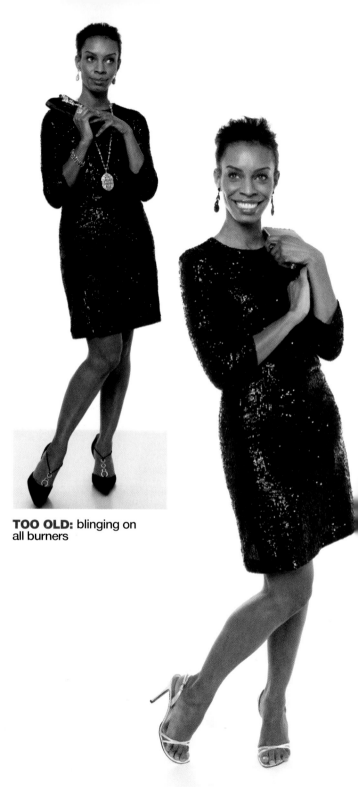

TOO OLD: blinging on all burners

JUST RIGHT: understated elegance, so Y&H

flattering and elongating worn with a low neckline. A chunkier choker style often works well to break up the expanse of skin bared in a strapless dress. Beware of those big estate jewels that "the queen" would wear. For a *Today* show segment on diamonds, I interviewed Neil Lane, jeweler to young Hollywood. He told me that those "dowager duchess" pieces lay too heavy on the neck and that it's younger to wear diamonds that have movement, that are swingy, fun, and more casual. Dowager duchess pieces will surely age you, as no one young could possibly afford them!

■ **Earrings:** You'll need to think about your hair when you're trying on earrings. And size does matter. Huge, heavy chandeliers dripping from your earlobes say OL unless you have a long, slender neck worth calling attention to. A better bet is shorter chandeliers or a simple drop. If you prefer studs, go for ones you can actually see. Again, better to wear a two-carat authentic-looking fake than a real diamond chip. Whenever we showed models in "diamond studs" on the *Today* show, they were wearing two-carat lookers from Givenchy ($28).

■ **Bracelet:** This is one of those pieces where styles change nearly every season. If chunky is in, opt for one dramatic cuff or a couple of big bangles. Read the fashion magazines, and you'll know.

■ **Watch:** You'll want to wear either a fancy bracelet or a watch, not both. And if you decide to wear your watch, it should be a dressy evening one. Your everyday watch with leather or stainless band

Photo Op!

Here's one of many great ideas from stylist Genevieve Yraola. Have someone snap a few digital photos of you (from various angles, standing, sitting, and so on) all dressed up in your party outfit. "Treat it like a dress rehearsal," says Genevieve. "Looking at the photos will allow you to step outside yourself and really see what you look like." And it will help you to see if everything you've selected really does work together. Do it at least a few days before the event so that, if need be, you still have time to go out and buy new underwear (see chapter 16 for tips on the sleekest shapewear for evening), rethink your jewelry, or look for different shoes.

will kill your look. Dressy watches don't have to be expensive. Check out the collections from Anne Klein, Michael Kors, and Moschino at Bloomingdale's (less than $200).

■ **Rings:** Giant cocktail rings — fabulous fakes or the real thing — go in and out of style. When they're in, they can be a fun addition to an evening look. I wear an R. J. Graziano "yellow diamond" every day that everyone thinks is real!

THE FINISHING TOUCHES: EVENING BAGS, SHOES, WRAPS

Even if you've picked out the most phenomenal dress and smashing jewelry to accessorize it, you can quickly blow the entire outfit if you overlook the impact of a stunning evening bag, sexy shoes, and a fashionable wrap.

■ **Evening bags:** Whether you choose a simple satin clutch or something with a jewel-encrusted clasp, your evening bag should be as dressy as the rest of your outfit. Have fun with it — it should complement, not match, your shoes and dress. *Please don't* go the kitschy route. Those little jeweled bags that are shaped like teddy bears or pieces of fruit can look adorable — on a sixteen-year-old.

■ **Shoes:** The simpler the dress, the fancier the shoes, and vice versa. Sexy heels are obviously the best choice, but don't go so high that you have to kick them off and walk around barefoot at the end of the party. If possible, keep your legs bare. (See chapter 17 for tips on stockings and other ways to dress up legs for evening.)

■ **Wraps and coats:** Ditch the been-there, done-that pashmina in favor of something fresher. The cool wrap changes from season to season. Right now, wraps made from lace or brocade look Y&H. A cropped little jacket — in velvet, satin, or jacquard — is also a cool option. Real or faux fur stoles make a dramatic statement, but nothing says OL faster than a big, bearlike mink coat. If you're going to wear a fur (or fake fur) coat, make sure it's styled to fit close to the body and long enough to cover your dress. The exception is a cropped, above-the-waist fur jacket, which looks sensational with a long gown.

FOLLOW THE
THREE-BLING RULE

Now, some fashion math. You need to count up your bling, because you are allowed only three bling points. But the equation is not *quite* as simple as one, two, three. Here are a few of Genevieve's evening equations.

■ Sparkly dress (2 bling points) + earrings (1 bling) − necklace = 3 bling points

■ Black dress (0 bling) + bold necklace (1 bling) + cocktail ring (1 bling) + shoes *or* bag (1 bling) − big earrings = 3 bling points

■ Jeweled cuff bracelet (1 bling) + shimmery metallic sandals (1 bling) + chandelier earrings (1 bling) − watch = 3 bling points

■ Dramatic upswept do (1 bling) + drop earrings (1 bling) + bracelet *or* ring (1 bling) − necklace = 3 bling points

Remember that location matters: You don't want to use two bling points in close proximity. Don't do a big necklace *and* big earrings. Don't do an oversized cocktail ring *and* a bracelet. Don't do a bracelet *and* a jeweled watch. Once the bling is hiding too much of you or your dress, you've overdone it. The goal is to look effortlessly elegant, not as if you're hiding beneath a shield of shiny armor.

HIGH, MEDIUM, AND LOW MAINTENANCE . . . EVENING HAIR AND MAKEUP

Your hair and makeup should be considered another accessory, and the same rule of not overdoing it applies. In fact, Isaac Mizrahi maintains that it's much more modern to "do" one or the other: hair *or* makeup. In other words, if you choose an elaborate hairstyle, tone down the makeup. If you have serious makeup, go with casual hair. Otherwise, you're going to look OL. Also, stay away from a schoolmarmish, tight bun and shimmery makeup. Although both can look chic on a twenty-year-old, they tend to be aging.

HIGH: For a big event, nothing is more fun than putting yourself in the hands of the professionals. So if you've got the time, money, and inclination, book appointments for a haircut, color, and styling, as well as a makeup application. Just remember to leave one or the other looking unfussy.

MEDIUM: Do your own makeup, but treat yourself to a professional blow-out. Whether you leave your hair down or put it up, it will be guaranteed to look fantastic. If you wear contacts, try colored contact lenses for a fun way to enhance your look and really make your eyes pop.

LOW: Do your own makeup *and* your hair, but give yourself extra time since this is a special event. Blow-dry and style your hair rather than wash and go; bring out the flat iron (or curling iron). Ramp up your usual makeup routine to include some evening extras, such as individual false eyelashes to make yours look even more lush and flirty.

FRAGRANCE:
READ BEFORE YOU SPRAY

It's so OL to have your fragrance enter the room before you do. Like all good things, perfume should be used in moderation. But some older women have the unfortunate habit of dousing themselves in so much scent that it takes over the room. And then there are the fragrances that scream OL. To get the word on how to choose a Y&H scent and the newer way to wear it, I talked scents with Yves de Chiris, a renowned fragrance creator responsible for some of the biggest launches of our time, whose family has been in the biz in France since 1768 (and even had their nose in Chanel No. 5!).

TOO DONE: Felicity Huffman in 2006

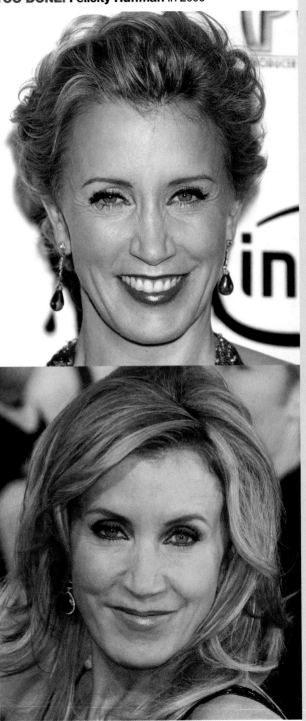

JUST RIGHT: loose hair, softer makeup, in 2007

145

Q&A on Fragrance

How not to O.D. on fragrance?
It's much better to spritz more often with less fragrance. That way, you renew the experience — just as you would touch up your makeup. Use three or four quick spritzes. Your skin will alter the scent, so it's better to spray it onto your hair, your underwear, or your blouse. It won't stain, and there's too little alcohol in it to damage your hair.

Is it possible to have a signature scent without seeming dated?
Avoid the mass brands and find a scent that's not as well known. Shop boutiques for those cultish, niche brands such as Jo Malone, Creed, and Fresh. It's not really the fragrance that communicates "old-fashioned," but the way it is worn. A rich Oriental scent worn by an older, overly made-up woman will signal old-fashioned. The same scent worn by someone who looks chic and young will signal sophistication.

Should you have a signature scent or mix it up?
Have a wardrobe of three or four scents — the fragrance equivalents of a pair of jeans, a chic suit, and a sexy cocktail dress — and choose which one you wear when just as you choose an outfit.

What scents would you consider "grandma" fragrances?
It's interesting that when a fragrance becomes a classic, it's also considered old-fashioned. A fragrance that has become a classic is a work of art, and if you choose to wear one because you like it, don't be ashamed of it. That said, here are a few alternatives to some classics if you want to try something different and more modern.

The classic: Shalimar
The alternatives: Obsession, Dune, Ambre Extrême, Must de Cartier

The classic: Chanel No. 5
The alternatives: Rive Gauche, White Linen, Anna Sui, Dream Angels Divine

The classic: Fracas
The alternatives: Marc Jacobs, Jo Malone Gardenia, Annick Goutal Passion

The classic: L'Air du Temps
The alternatives: Red Door, Bulgari Pour Femme, Beautiful

How long will a bottle of perfume keep its scent?
If you keep it cool (even in the refrigerator), a bottle will last about two years. Strong sunlight or heat will cause it to deteriorate more quickly.

They Do Evening Just Right

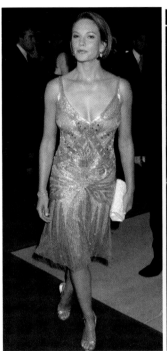

Diane Lane

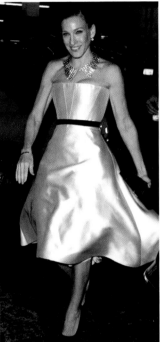

Sarah Jessica Parker

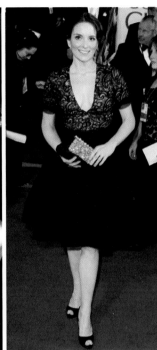

Tina Fey

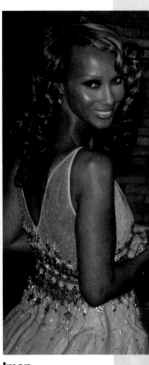

Iman

YOUR BLACK-TIE PROP KIT

As we learned in Girl Scouts: Be Prepared! Assemble your "prop kit" in your spare (ha, ha) time, and keep it in a plastic bin in your closet marked "Black Tie."

- Jeweled evening bag
- Tiny compact
- Tiny pen
- Tiny comb
- Altoids
- Light nail color
- Lip gloss
- Fancy bracelet

- Gel petals (for nipple show-through; see chapter 16)
- Convertible bra
- Dressy watch
- Leg spray
- Heel helpers (see chapter 18)

Did You Know That

A spritz of pink grapefruit will make you appear six years younger to men? A recent study by the Smell & Taste Treatment and Research Foundation in Chicago concluded that in the presence of the smell of pink grapefruit, women appear to be six years younger than their real age. One of the best scents with a grapefruit top note: Jo Malone Grapefruit Cologne (3.4 fl. oz.), $95; available at select Neiman Marcus and Saks Fifth Avenue stores or Jo Malone Shops, jomalone.com. It also comes in a delicious bath oil, shower gel, body lotion, body crème, and home candle! Why not smell young, too?

THE THREE-BLING RULE WHEN DRESSING FOR EVENING

LEARN TO LOVE
SHAPEWEAR
16

NOTHING AGES YOU LIKE ...
GRANNY PANTS ... VPL ... GIRDLE LEGS ... SAUSAGING ... MUFFIN TOPS ... SPILLAGE ... BACK FAT ... SAGGY BREASTS ... MASSIVE BREASTS ... A UNIBOOB

When I was twenty, my lingerie drawer was packed with teeny, flimsy things exploding with color: fluorescent pink, hot orange, and acid green bikini undies; red and purple bustiers; a cobalt blue lacy camisole; a silver lamé garter belt; and if the bra fit, it was there in every color. Now my lingerie drawer is basically nude and black, and reserved for only the most powerful high-performance weapons designed to help the modern woman win her daily war against droopage. To be honest, one lingerie drawer isn't enough to contain my ever-expanding arsenal. My armory is housed in one half of an enormous armoire organized into easy-to-grab-in-the-morning bins: bras, panties, bike shorts and leg shapers, bodysuits and slips, opaque stockings, leggings, fishnets. Of course, I still own a few flimsy, sexy pieces of intimate apparel, but they don't get out much anymore. Even on a Saturday night, I'm one hundred times more likely to reach for a reliable pair of Spanx Tight End Reversible Tights with Tummy Control to wear under my sweater dress than a garter belt or the pair of sheer black stay-up stockings I haven't worn since the first George Bush was in the White House.

Here's the point: the older we get, the more we demand of our underwear. Once you hit thirty, sexy alone doesn't cut it. Our first layer of armor in the battle against aging has to be super-supportive. What lies beneath our great jeans, jersey wrap dresses, and especially red-carpet-worthy gowns are fashion's unsung heroes — the hardest-working pieces in our wardrobes, those miracle workers called shapewear. They lift! They smooth! They mold! They shape! They minimize! They hide ten pounds! They take inches off (so you can now get into that sheath you thought you couldn't zip up anymore)! You'd be surprised how shapewear can open up new wardrobe possibilities. And that's not all. Awesome advances in fabrication and technology lift and separate this new breed of lightweight, high-performance microfibers from OL girdles, making them comfy enough to wear all day and all night. Pity our poor mothers, who had to suck it up in painful corsets, maiming themselves in the name of fashion. How lucky we are to have soft, pliable, heavily injected with Lycra or spandex body shapers, waist whittlers, bike shorts, footless panty hose, control thongs, slips, and camis ready to make our bodies look thinner, smoother, tighter, smaller, higher, sexier. Whatever the next style challenge, bring it on! We're ready!

EVEN GWYNETH WEARS IT
As you can probably tell, I love shapewear. I believe in shapewear. Shapewear has changed my life! And it can do the same for you. Sara Blakely, the founder of the ever-expanding Spanx line, knows the feeling: "Women tell me all the time,

'I feel more confident in my Spanx.' 'I don't feel properly dressed unless I'm in my Spanx.' 'I don't leave the house without Spanx.' " There you have it: shapewear transcends the physical. Is there a woman alive who doesn't want to be in control?

In the right shapewear, anything is possible, and not only for those of us who are lifetime members of Weight Watchers, with a constant eye on the scale. As we age, even the thinnest among us have areas of soft flesh — affectionately referred to as back fat, muffin tops, Buddha bellies, saddle-bags, and various other parts that need to be, well, managed. So don't think of shapewear as underwear for plus-sizers only. Even size 2s want to feel as if they are in control of their bodies. Make that especially size 2s. It's now a given that every woman of style wears shapewear — from the cast of *Desperate Housewives* to Katie Couric to Oprah to Gwyneth Paltrow. Yes, even Gwyneth has owned up to the fact that she wore two pairs of Spanx bike shorts post-baby. Love her for confirming what we suspected all along: all the Hollywood girls do it.

By the end of this chapter, you'll know exactly what to buy for every bulge on your body. But first, your lingerie drawer needs a makeover.

ONLY "GOOD" LINGERIE FROM NOW ON

When you're rushing out the door in the morning, you don't want to waste precious minutes sorting through underwear. Do yourself a favor: Get rid of every bra, panty, and shaper that's not "good." You know what I mean: we all classify our underwear as "good" or "bad," depending on how long it's languished in the drawer and how well it fits. On a day you have to dress to impress, you'll select your "good" underwear. On a day you're hanging around the house or just having the gardener come over, you'll opt for the old, worn-out bra or those nasty OL "granny pants" (aka big, unsupportive bloomers that cover not only your derriere but also most of your lower back and stomach). Ugh! The goal here is to purge your drawer of the "bad" so that anything you grab from this day forward will be "good," because you're only going to look fabulous from now on — even if it's just for you or the gardener. (If you recall, during the first season of *Desperate Housewives*, Gabrielle wore only her best for the gardener!)

Plan this makeover for a weekend afternoon when you have a couple of hours to yourself and can shut the door, try on, and look in the mirror.

1. Take your lingerie drawer and dump the contents out on your bed.

2. Separate it into categories: shapers (aka girdles), bras, panties, slips.

3. Take all the "good" in the bra, panty, and shapewear categories and place them back in the drawer. All slips that aren't shapewear slips get the slip, because old-fashioned, unsupportive slips are so OL. Sexy, underwear-as-outerwear, vintage slips are totally Y&H and should be hung in your closet so they're top of mind.

4. Toss the remaining pieces into the trash. If they're relatively new and clean, you can assuage your guilt by donating them to a wonderful women's organization such as Bottomless Closet (bottomlesscloset.org) or Dress for Success (dressforsuccess.org). Try on every piece that you have trouble tossing and take the "to toss or not to toss test" found in each lingerie category. You'll find it's easier to say good-bye when you know the reason you must liberate yourself from this no-good piece that doesn't deserve to live in your drawer, let alone embrace your body.

If you answer yes to any of the following questions, take a deep breath, exhale, and toss. Aaah!

Shapers

Before shapewear, there were girdles. If you still own any old-fashioned "foundation garments," disown these archetypal relics ASAP. Shapewear companies are constantly improving on fit, fashion, function, and technology, launching new styles as often as five times a year. There's absolutely no reason to keep torture wear, since a comfier solution is definitely out there. For this test, try on all girdles, bike shorts, waist whittlers, and body and leg shapers under a pair of revealing white pants.

- Is it a struggle to get into it?
- Is it difficult to breathe once you're in there?
- Is it impossible to forget that you have it on?
- Is it showing visible signs of wear and tear?
- Is it so stretched out that it's lost its function?
- Do you feel as if you would be just as shapely naked?
- Do you have bulges of skin where the bands meet your body?
- Are the leg bands visible when you're wearing pants?
- Is the fabric so bulky that it's actually adding weight?
- Do the seams — front, back, or sides — show through the pants?
- Are there annoying hooks, ties, or zipper closures?
- Do the bands cut off circulation to the point where you feel as if you're wearing a tourniquet?
- Is it white?

Bras

Try on each bra and look in a mirror. To get the full picture, slip on a white T-shirt or sweater over the bra to analyze shape and show-through.

- Is it shabby?
- Is it stretched out?
- Do you spill out of the top, bottom, or sides?
- Is it so tight that it gives you a smashed-in uniboob?
- Is there puckering in the cups?
- Is there lace show-through?
- Is there nipple show-through?
- Is the underwire poking out or stabbing you?
- With the straps at their tightest, do you hang too low? (See "The Saggy Boobs Test" later in this chapter.)
- Does it feel scratchy?
- Is it in any way uncomfortable?
- Is it too young-looking — i.e., would a teenager wear it?
- Does it look matronly — i.e., would your grandma wear it?
- Is the color too garish?
- Would you be embarrassed to be seen wearing it in the locker room?

Still Have a Hard Time Tossing?

I know it's hard to part with old friends, so if you're still not sure that your old lingerie is "good" for everyday, here's my pain-free solution. Get a plastic bin and label it with a sticker that says "B LINGERIE" and the date. Stash the bin high on a closet shelf or under the bed — somewhere without easy access. Make a deal with yourself: any B piece that you don't seek out within one year from the date on the sticker gets tossed.

Panties

Don't waste your time trying on granny pants. Even if you are a granny, you don't want to dress like one, so all big bloomers must exit your life now. (Or if you can stand looking at them again, recycle them as dust rags.) From this day forward, promise yourself that your lingerie drawer will have only panties that are certified Y&H. To assess all other panties, try on each pair and check out the rear view in a three-way mirror. To assess VPL potential, pull on a pair of white pants.

■ **Would you be horrified to let the ER team see you in this?**

■ **Does it look shabby?**

■ **Is it stretched out? Threadbare? Pilled?**

■ **Is there a stray strand of elastic sticking out?**

■ **Are the leg bands digging into your thighs?**

■ **Is the waistband so tight that you get love handles or a muffin top?**

■ **Is there sausaging — obvious indentation above or below the elastic bands?**

■ **Is the seat saggy?**

■ **Is it 100 percent cotton without any stretch?**

■ **Is the crotch anything but 100 percent cotton?**

■ **Does it give you VPL on the sides? In the rear? On the top or bottom?**

■ **Is it so sheer that even a Brazilian bikini wax would show through?**

■ **Is it too young-looking — i.e., embellished with words, arrows, hearts, dogs, or other animals?**

■ **Would your mom wear it?**

■ **Is the color too crazy?**

■ **Is it uncomfortable in any way?**

■ **Would an exotic dancer perform in it?**

DESIGN YOUR SHAPEWEAR SHOPPING LIST

You'll save yourself time, not to mention drama, if you know what pieces are best before you hit the stores. Check out the list of Brilliant Buys and assess the body issues you need to manage. And if you have a certain outfit in your closet that would look a lot better if only you had the right underpinnings, bring it with you. "I don't care whether you are a [size] 0, 2, 4, or 10, every woman has that one item in her closet that she just doesn't wear," says Sara Blakely of Spanx, who could never find the right underwear for her white pants before she invented Spanx. If it's a long evening gown, you might not want the hassle of toting around a cumbersome garment bag. A better strategy, then, is to buy a few items, try them on at home, and return the ones you don't want. Just make sure the store accepts returns before you go there.

Let's Go Shapewear Shopping

Before you leave the house, go online to find the brands and styles your store carries. Retailers are

Rules for Drama-Free Shapewear Shopping

1. Go solo. Squeezing into these pieces is humiliating enough. You don't need to perform in front of company.

2. Allow yourself a good two hours in the dressing room. You don't want to be rushed, and you don't want to have to come back to finish the job.

3. Get there early in the morning or late in the evening. That's when the store is quiet and you'll get the attention you need when you're standing naked in the dressing room pleading for another size. Liz Hosofar, divisional merchandise manager for intimate apparel at Bloomingdale's, suggests making an appointment with a fitter.

4. Don't shop during a sale, when all hell breaks loose. There's nothing that kills your appetite for shopping quite like standing in a long line waiting for a dressing room.

5. If you find yourself in a store with lying mirrors, dingy lighting, skimpy spaces, or inattentive help, go elsewhere.

---

constantly dropping and adding collections to their assortments, because the better stores want exclusives on the newest, latest, and greatest. If you have your sights set on the Spanx slip, for instance, go online to see if it's still at a Bloomingdale's near you. Of course, you can avoid the stores completely and shop online in your bathrobe, but for your virgin shopping trip, it's best to seek professional help. You need a proper fitting by a pro in a specialty shop or the lingerie department of a well-stocked department store such as Bloomingdale's or Nordstrom. She will put a tape measure around your waist and tell you if you're an S, M, or L. But do shop for your shapewear replacements online at a site such as barenecessities.com, which carries a wide range of brands. It's a breeze once you know your styles and sizes.

SMART SHOPPING TIP #1: Get nude, not white. Even under a white T-shirt, nude looks better. But buy a few pieces of black to wear under dark fabrics; it won't show dirt as much and get as shabby-looking. When traveling for a family party, I once made the mistake of bringing only a white bra with me. Let me tell you, white under black jersey is not a pretty sight. Would you like to see the photos?

So that this won't ever happen to you, don't even buy white shapewear. You don't need it.

SMART SHOPPING TIP #2: Some lines, such as Spanx and Maidenform Flexees, offer a have-it-your-way menu in terms of compression. So you can choose how you like your shapewear: light, moderate, or firm.

- **Light** (or everyday control) smoothes bulges and protects you against VPL.
- **Moderate** stops jiggling.
- **Firm** can actually take off inches.

The trade-off, of course, is comfort for control. Your comfort level decreases as control increases. Too much compression in the bust, for instance, and you feel as if you're having a mammogram all day. Remember that compression alone isn't going to get you gorgeous. In the bust and bum, you need to be shaped, also, to avoid uniboob and bubble butt. If you're already in good shape, you may not need "firm" shapewear day in and day out, but you'll want some in the drawer, ready when you need to pull out the heavy artillery.

SHAPEWEAR FROM TOP TO BOTTOM

As our generation expands, so does the shape-wear industry. There are the pioneer brands — such as Spanx, Donna Karan Intimates, Wacoal, Body Wrap, Maidenform, Nancy Ganz, and Hanes — and the newer kids on the block — such as Vera Wang, Sassybax, Cass and Co., and Lipo in a Box — all competing for control of your body. After weeks of dressing room research, I've come up with a list of brilliant buys I absolutely swear by, with two important caveats: (1) What's best for me may not be best for you, so use this list for starters and prepare to do some exploration on your own. (2) By the time you read this, some styles may have been discontinued and replaced by new and improved versions. Ask your savvy sales associate for the update.

TO SMOOTH BACK FAT AND EVERYTHING DOWN TO YOUR WAIST

Flexees One Fabulous Body Everyday Control Camisole, style 77320, $25.50, and **Flexees** One Fabulous Body Everyday Control Camisole (with bra), style 77390, $35; maidenform.com

If you can get away without wearing a bra, choose the first cami in S, M, or L in beige or black. If you need a bra, the second one comes in molded-cup bra sizes. With or without a bra, this nylon and 12 percent Lycra cami feels like a dream. Wear it under sweaters, blouses, and dresses, and watch those little pouches of fat under your armpits inching toward your back disappear. Plus, it smoothes your entire midriff so that it's roll-free. The Flexees beat out every other cami I road-tested for two reasons: (1) The compression is comfortable. I don't feel as if I'm in a straitjacket. (2) It's cropped short and doesn't come down all the way to my mid-thigh, like some of these do. Petites don't need all that extra fabric bunching up around the hips.

TO PREVENT BUDDHA BELLY, SLIMMING YOUR STOMACH SOUTH OF YOUR BRA BAND TO MID-THIGH

Lipo in a Box High Waist Brief with Legs, style 46821, $40; lipoinabox.com

I recently wore this to a holiday party, and it saved the outfit. I was wearing a gold sequined cardigan with a tight, stretchy, white T-shirt underneath and jeans. Without this lifesaver, I had a roll from my bra band to the top of the jeans. After I put this on, everything was smooth, chic, and under control. I never thought I needed a high-waisted piece, but I do.

TO SLIM YOUR ENTIRE STOMACH SOUTH OF YOUR BRA BAND TO MID-CALF; UNDER PANTS WITH OPEN-TOE SHOES

Spanx High-Falutin' Footless, style 160, $28; 888-806-7311 or spanx.com; Bloomingdale's, 800-232-1854

It's the newest incarnation of the famous footless panty hose that started the Spanx revolution. This style now goes all the way up to your bra band, so you're covered from under your bust to mid-thigh — no spillage! Footless Spanx also comes in Hipnotic for under low-rise pants and skirts (style 098, $26 at spanx.com).

TO WHITTLE YOUR MIDDLE

Maidenform Control It! Sexy Waistnipper Brief, style 12419, $25; maidenform.com

For those Scarlett O'Hara moments, this piece comes up to your bra band to give you your best shot at an hourglass waistline while slimming your lower tummy, too. There are no hooks and eyes to fiddle with, and it gives you a completely smooth line because it doesn't end below the belly button. Just FYI, if your thighs need slimming too, this is not for you because the bottom half is a brief, not a bike short, so it's strictly for middle management.

TO SLIM YOUR HIPS AND LOWER TUMMY AND BOOST YOUR DERRIERE
Donna Karan Body Perfect Level 1 Mid-Thigh, $30; Nordstrom, nordstrom.com

I have been a fan of Donna Karan's bike shorts for years because they're made of the lightest microfibers and hold in without hurt — comfortable enough for daily wear. The leg bands are thin, so you can wear them with total confidence under pants. For more control, there is also a Level 2 for $32.

TO SLIM YOUR LOWER TUMMY
Donna Karan Control Brief, $42; Neiman Marcus, neimanmarcus.com

These can be your go-to panties for days when your thighs can take care of themselves. They're 95 percent nylon and 5 percent spandex, so the comfort is there.

TO SLIM YOUR LOWER TUMMY WHILE WEARING JUST A THONG
Control It! by Maidenform Firm Control Thong, style 12412, $19; maidenform.com

Control thongs, a genius way to expose your butt cheeks yet suck in your tummy, aren't available in every line, so if you love thongs, this one's for you. It's tagless, too, which means that the care info is printed on the fabric instead of a hanging label that may cause a bump under the clingiest fabrics.

A Bit of Shapewear Herstory

Spanx founder Sara Blakely had all but given up on the idea of creating the first footless panty hose after failing to convince the male-dominated hosiery industry that women wanted footless so that they could have the control of panty hose plus the freedom to wear sandals. She was in a Detroit hotel on a business trip when she turned on the TV and saw Oprah telling viewers how she cuts off her panty hose at the feet to wear under long skirts with sandals. Sara didn't know until later that I was the guest that Oprah was telling her panty hose secret to! This "aha" moment for Sara gave her the confidence to keep pushing, which is why Footless is Sara's first and favorite piece of Spanx.

TO SMOOTH YOU OUT ALL OVER IN A HIP SLIP
Spanx Hide & Sleek Full Slip, style 060A, $72; Strapless Full Slip, style 077A, $72; and Half Slip, style 054A, $52; spanx.com or 888-806-7311

Meet the Y&H slip (see next page). These cool smoothers replace all those OL ones you just tossed out. They not only erase all visible lines, but they also have double-layer compression to still all those wobbly bits under light or clingy fabrics. If you love slips, check out all three tagless styles. These could be the last slips you ever buy.

TO CONTROL YOUR BULGES AND JIGGLES
FROM YOUR BOOBS TO YOUR CALVES
Lipo in a Box Capri Bodysuit with underwire,
style 46301, or without underwire, style 46303,
$86; Lipo in a Box, lipoinabox.com

For all-over control, this shaper really does feel like
a second skin — a triumph since most of these
all-encompassing numbers are uncomfortable. I
prefer the underwire — more shape and support.
Big plus: Both pieces have gusseted openings
for bathroom ease. You don't want a one-piece

that you have to take off from the straps down
every time you visit the loo. All-over body slimmers
ensure there is no spillage anywhere on your body
and no seams to break the line of your clothing.
This is the thing to buy before your next high
school reunion.

LIFT OFF! PULLING YOURSELF UP BY YOUR BRA STRAPS

No shapewear shopping list would be complete
without a supportive new bra. Now that may seem
like an obvious statement to you, but the intimate
apparel biz does not consider bras shapewear
but rather lingerie. Which is why some department
stores have shapewear departments separate from
lingerie departments. As a shopper, this makes
me crazy, because I have to get dressed, walk to
another department, find another sales associate, stand in line for another dressing room, and
undress yet again. Thanks a lot, guys! And I do
mean guys, because the intimate apparel business
has traditionally been run by men who clearly don't
realize that when your breasts start to sag, a garment that can place two pendulous pieces of flesh
back into their original upright positions is the most
important shapewear item a woman can buy, right
up there on the list of Top 10 Things That Make You
Look Y&H. The heavy lifting accomplished by this
relatively small swatch of fabric is nothing short of
miraculous. The right bra is your low-maintenance
breast-lift. For that, we must now pay homage to its
masterful design and give the bra its proper boost.

Look Ten Years Younger and Ten Pounds Thinner — with the Right Bra!

When was the last time you were fitted for a bra? If
you're like most women, you're wearing the wrong
bra size right now. We've all heard the alarming
stats that either 70 or 85 percent of us (depending
on the study) are walking around in a bra that's too
small or too big. Full disclosure: I was in the wrong
size when I started researching this chapter. Why
do our breasts fluctuate so? When we're young,

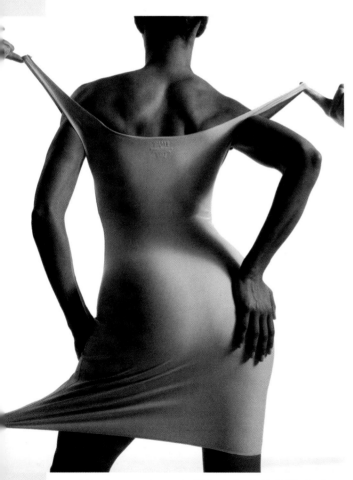

JUST RIGHT: Spanx's Hide & Seek Full Slip is the
hip slip that stills all those wobbly bits.

The Saggy Boobs Test

Using a metal tape measure, stand in front of a mirror and measure the distance from the top of your shoulder to the crease in your elbow. Put on the new bra. If your nipple resides halfway between your shoulder and elbow, you have a winner. For larger breasts, look for a 60/40 split (a 40 percent lift from the elbow). This is an eye-opener! Most of us wear bras that don't give the proper uplift.

our breasts are firm, because they consist of more glandular tissue than fat. As we age, due to estrogen loss at menopause, the glandular tissue shrivels up and is replaced by fat. Now that our breasts are mostly fat, they're softer, more pendulous, often larger, and very sensitive to changes in weight. (Who said that getting older is fun?) That's why bra experts suggest getting refitted for a bra at least once a year, or if you experience any of the following:

- A five- to seven-pound weight loss or gain

- A change in diet or exercise program

- Menopause

- Breast surgery, including implants, reduction, or lift

Let's Go Bra Shopping

The best thing you can do for yourself is surrender to the tape measure of a professional bra fitter at a good department store or specialty shop. Don't bother trying to determine your correct bra size yourself with the various mathematical tables available all over the Web, because they aren't always accurate. My bra pro showed me that according to the chart, I would be less than a size A (and I know that's not the case).

Expect to bring ten or more different styles into the fitting room with you. You have to do a lot

of test-driving before you find your dream bra (it's like dating). Even if it's your size, it might not be the right cut for you. And sizes are not consistent; even within the same brand, you may have to go up or down in cup or band size in different styles. Wear a tight, light-colored sweater or T-shirt so you can give the bra the ultimate test under clothes. When you think you've found your dream bra, make sure that all three elements — cups, band, straps — are supporting you in every way (see below).

The second-best thing you can do for yourself is to determine whether a new bra is hoisting you high enough. This is what will make you appear ten pounds thinner, instantly creating the appearance of a longer and leaner torso by giving you extra inches where your breasts used to be. Breasts that hang long and low are so OL! Whether you're in the dressing room or in front of the mirror at home, whip out a tape measure and take the saggy boobs test.

The right cup: You want a cup that's roomy enough to house your entire breast. What looks OL is flesh that hangs over the top, under the band, or out the sides. In a fitted sweater or T-shirt, you want to look smoothly Y&H, not like you actually have four breasts, counting the two fleshy pockets poking out of the top. The most common mistake women make when shopping for a bra is shoving too-large breasts into too-shallow cups. A cup is the right size when it encases and lies flat on the entire breast without extra material or air. If you're large breasted, the cup should also pull your breasts off

... the average bra size in America has increased from 34B to 36C.

your rib cage without flattening them out. You want your breasts to have a nice, rounded slope, not look like a shelf.

Don't feel bad if you need to up the cup. Once we hit forty, many of us need a bigger cup size. Donna Lennon, a bra specialist for twenty-five years who runs Drawer Full of Lingerie in Boca Raton, Florida, reports that most women have no problem increasing their band size but are loath to increase their cup size. "I cannot tell you the number of women who come in and say 'I'm a 34C,' and they're a 34DD," says Donna. "They assume they're smaller than they are, and they do not want to be refitted. They just want to buy the same thing over and over again." If it makes you feel any better, American women are collectively getting bigger. According to a study by Bali, the average bra size has increased from 34B to 36C over the last fifteen years. Good news for the bigger busted: specialty shops such as Donna's now carry sizes up to DDDD.

Just FYI, most women have one breast that's larger than the other. You should always fit the larger breast, and you can use a silicone pad, if necessary, to fill out the smaller cup (and prevent show-through, too). Check out the Smart Cups by Connie Elder ($25; Lipo in a Box, lipoinabox.com). **The right band:** Think of it as the unsung hero of the bra triumvirate. The band — not the straps — should do most of the heavy lifting. You want a band that feels snug (not tight) and doesn't dig into your flesh, causing it to seep over the band (aka OL back fat). Some women hike up the band,

hoping to prevent back fat, but actually they're creating it. For a Y&H look, make sure the back band is in the proper position: level across the narrow part of your back beneath your shoulder blades. Seem low? Maybe it's because you've been wearing it wrong for so long. When trying on a new bra, always fasten the band on the middle or loosest hook. With wear, the band will stretch, and you'll need the tightest hook to compensate.

The right straps: If your bra can stay up even without straps, bra-vo. Straps are supposed to do only 20 percent of the work, so if you're constantly pulling yourself up by your bra straps to get lift-off, you're not in the right bra. If unhooking your bra and saying "Aaah!" is one of the first things you do when you get home, chances are you're not in the right bra. If the straps are so tight that they dig in and leave OL red marks or indentations on your skin, try thicker straps and padded straps. Another sign that you're not wearing the right bra? Needing to yank up the straps in the back with a safety pin. (How Y&H are you going to look when the pin unfastens and stabs you in the back?) Yet another sign that you're in the wrong bra: having to go to a tailor to get the straps shortened. Sorry, but you still haven't found a bra that fits (see Brilliant Buys).

YOUR BRA WARDROBE

We've all been there: rushing to get dressed for a special event, you realize that you don't have the right bra for the occasion. To make sure that you're always equipped, here's a cheat sheet of some brands that do each category of bra best. All of the bras listed are certifiably Y&H. All of these performance (nonsexy) bras have soft, molded, seamless cups made of lightweight, springy, modern microfibers that will make your breasts so happy, you'll barely remember you have a bra on. (OL bras are traditionally white, with stiff, scratchy, cotton cups that may include perforations, topstitching, obvious seams, and nerdy decorative details such as flowers, birds, or butterflies.) What colors to buy? Nude and black. The most popular bra color is white, but even nude looks better under a white shirt. How many bras do you need? The average American woman has eight, wears only four. The lowest-maintenance woman needs a minimum of three bras: one to wear, one to wash, one on standby. The rest of us need at least three in the essential T-shirt bra category, at least one that's an enhancer or minimizer, a strapless, a deep-V, and a sexy for show — which totals seven bras. Add a couple of sports bras, and you're at nine.

1. Best Everyday Bra for Under T-Shirts

■ *For bigger busts:* **Le Mystere** Renaissance Dream Tisha Bra (34C–38G), $68; Bloomingdale's. The T-shirt bra of my dreams — like I've never been lifted before!

■ *For middle-size busts:* **Wacoal** i-Bra Contour Bra (32B–38D), $50; Nordstrom. Everyone loves this stitchless, tagless, laser-cut bra, Oprah included.

■ *For smaller busts:* **Playtex** "Thank Goodness It Fits" Santoni Light Lined SoCup Bra (32A–38C), $25; Kohl's, 800-564-5740; onehanesplace.com. Even in hot colors, there is no show-through. And it's the rare T-shirt bra offered in half sizes.

2. Best Cleavage Enhancer: Victoria's Secret

Angels Secret Embrace (32A–38D), $48; Victoria's Secret, 800-411-5116 or victoriassecret.com. Who needs implants when these pads, placed on the outside of each cup, push breasts inward for maximum cleavage?

3. Best Minimizer: Chantelle Volupte Smooth

Minimizer, style 2361 (up to size 38G), $68; Bloomingdale's. Who would ever guess what lies beneath? Takes you down a cup size — or two.

4. Best Strapless: Le Mystere Dream Shame-

less Strapless (32C–40G), $62; Bloomingdale's or barenecessities.com. You don't feel as if you're compromising uplift for straplessness.

5. Best for Deep-V, Halter Back, Racer Back:

Natori Underneath Sheer Mesh Ultralight Convertible Contour in Café (32A–36DD), $48; Nordstrom, 888-282-6060; barenecessities.com. If you love to wear low-cut sweaters and dresses, this bra lets you dive an inch and a half deeper than a regular bra — with a clear plastic strip between cups.

GENIUS BRA EXTRAS

1. To prevent nipple show-through: Fashion

Forms Gel Petals, $15; lingeriesolutions.com. Forget peeling back the old paper or fabric breast petals. The modern way to prevent show-through is with silicone, nude gel petals that stick to your nipples without bunching up and can be worn up to twenty-five times.

2. To prevent strap slippage: Fashion Forms

Strap Mate, $5.50; lingeriesolutions.com. At our age, showing your bra straps looks sloppy, not sexy. If you have a top that's cut skimpy and you don't have the right bra, tie your straps together in back with this nifty padded elastic band.

3. To hide straps: Fashion Forms Invisible Bra Straps, $8; lingeriesolutions.com. Another solution to strap slippage. Replace your straps with these clear stretchy ones.

4. To fill out a smaller cup: Smart Cups by Connie Elder, $25; lipoinabox.com

The Newer Way to . . .

Get Your Bra On

We've been doing it since the seventh grade, but many of us still don't know how to put on a bra correctly. I didn't. If your bra hooks in back, don't attach your bra in front and twist it around. This causes the band to stretch. Instead, just put it on with the hook in the back, feel around, and clasp it. It's tricky at first, but you'll get the hang of it. Then lean forward and scoop your breasts up and place them in the cups with your nipples centered. The tops of your breasts should look nice and full. Make sure your breasts are separated from each other. The squished-together look is so OL!

(PLEASE DON'T . . .)

Wear the same bra two days in a row. Rest your bra between wearings so it can "bounce back." Your bra actually relaxes with the warmth of your body, and if you wear the same bra constantly, it will lose its firmness.

WEAR THONGS: YES, YOU!

Now that you've rid yourself of granny pants, stock up on thongs. There's nothing wrong with wearing bikinis, briefs, or boy shorts, but thongs should be the staple of your Y&H panty collection — and the undies of choice when you're wearing a mid–low-rise jean. You need a low-rise panty to prevent VTE (visible thong exposure) and VPL at the same time. There are lots of beautiful microfiber thongs in the lingerie department, but the best are those with V-waists that dip lower in the front and back so you can quit playing peekaboo.

V-WAIST THONGS

Hanky Panky Low Rise Thong, style 4911, $18; Bloomingdale's
It's been called the most comfortable thong, so it's no wonder that this cult favorite is the best-selling thong at Bloomingdale's. Celebrities and Y&H women alike are addicted to the signature super-stretchy-lace rose pattern. It's so wildly popular that there's a mad rush for whatever the new color is. Don't worry about size; it comes only in one-size-fits-most. If you've never worn a thong before, start your collection here.

Jeanious Thongs by Barely There (S–XL), $9; onehanesplace.com
No need to go commando when you can buy Barely There for barely nothing. The slick yet silky nylon spandex won't bunch up or snag under your lowest jeans. So easy to buy online.

Other Lingerie To-Dos

✓ **Check Yourself Out from All Angles**

Invest in a good three-way mirror so you can see yourself as others see you — front, back, and sideways — before you walk out the door. You want to catch that glimpse of back fat or VPL before everyone else does — and fix it while you can.

✓ **Hand-Wash Your Shapewear**

Even if the label says that you can machine-wash, the machine cycle is too long, and the agitation is no friend to elasticity. (Think about it: Do manufacturers re-ally care how long your purchases last? They want you to buy new!) When hand-washing, use a delicate soap such as Ivory Snow or Forever New (designed specifically for lingerie). Always use cool water: it shocks the elastic into retaining its stretch and shape.

✓ **Buy Sexy Lingerie**

For sexy nights that call for something pretty, lacy, wild, and easy to remove. You don't want to make the mistake of Bridget Jones in *Bridget Jones's Diary.* She was so unprepared for hot sex with Daniel Cleaver that it took forever for him to remove her shapewear knickers. Nothing helps you get in the mood like drop-dead sexy lingerie. Every woman needs at least some go-to pieces in her drawer. If your cup size is on the small side, treat yourself to a racy, lacy bra and panty set. If money is no object, take your pick from the chicest name in lingerie, Italy's La Perla (figleaves .com). Or, check out Hanky Panky's new bras with matching panties ($48–$52 at Bloomingdale's) and Wacoal's Lost in Lace collection ($28–$48 at Nordstrom). The prettiest collection of larger size bras (36C–54H) and panties is by Fantasie of England at barenecessities .com. Don't fret about comfort here. If these pieces do what they're designed to, you won't be in them for long.

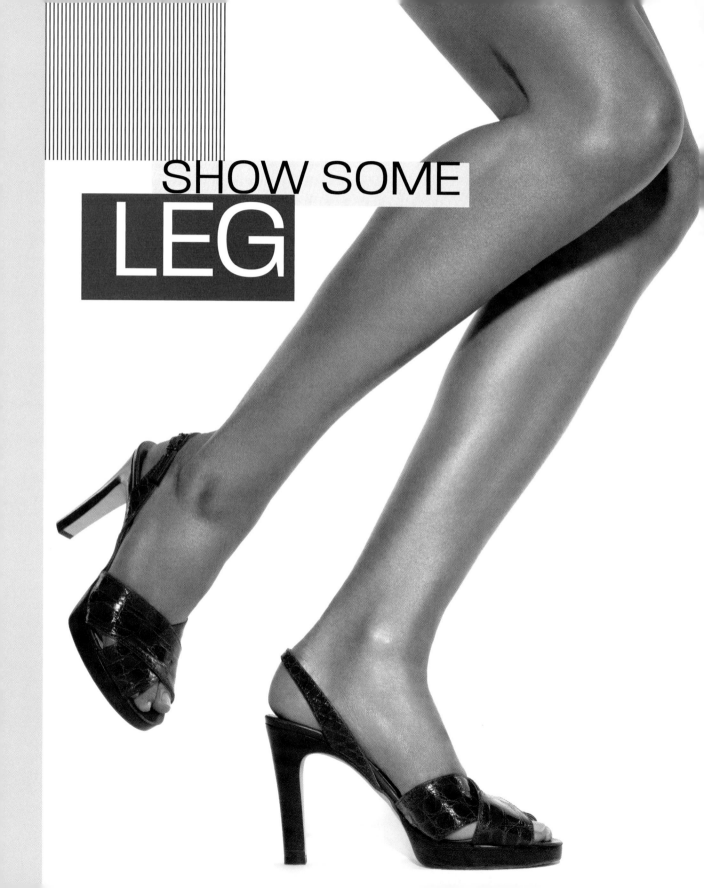

SHOW SOME
LEG

NOTHING AGES YOU LIKE . . .
THICK, FLESH-COLORED PANTY HOSE . . . STOCKINGS WITH REINFORCED TOES . . . STOCKINGS WITH SANDALS . . . WHITE STOCKINGS . . . HAIRY LEGS . . . FLAKY LEGS . . . PALE LEGS . . . NASTY-LOOKING VEINS

What you put on your legs is one of those decisions that immediately places you into either the OL or the Y&H category. Of course, it's easy to say that the most Y&H option is to show off gorgeous gams as much as possible. The problem with that theory is that it assumes you have gorgeous gams — and let's face it, many of us no longer do. If you've still got them, by all means flaunt them. There's nothing more Y&H than beautiful bare legs. For the rest of us, we need some fast and easy solutions for making our legs more bare-able.

But first, let's talk about stockings, because there are going to be occasions when you will feel the need to cover your legs. At this fashion moment, nude panty hose are the devil, and you should avoid them like the plague. Designer Isaac Mizrahi refers to legs in nude hose as "baloney legs," which gives you a pretty good idea of how awful he thinks they look. "Unless you're doing a kind of tongue-in-cheek thing about a stewardess in the sixties, which could be wonderful," he jokes. And unless you have a job today that requires nude hose as part of a uniform (and isn't there something you can do to change that?), wearing them says that you are seriously stuck in a time warp. Sure, I still have unopened packages of Donna Karan Nudes (which were, back in the

day, the only sheers worth wearing) in the back of my drawer because if there's one thing you can be sure of with fashion, it's that everything old is reinvented eventually. But, now, what should you wear on your legs?

ANYTHING BUT NUDE: LEGWEAR YOU CAN LOVE OR LEAVE

When in doubt, make sure whatever you put on your legs is subtle and sophisticated. You want your legs to look great, but they should meld seamlessly into your outfit, not scream for attention.

Opaques: These solid tights are a fabulous fall and winter solution. Just be careful not to buy those that are *too* thick, since they can make legs look bulky. Stock up on brown, black, gray, and navy lightweight opaques. The gold standard is Wolford's Velvet De Luxe Tights. Another genius option is Spanx Tight End Reversible Tights. They're black on one side and either brown or gray on the other (just turn them inside out), so you get two wearings for each washing, which is especially great for travel.

Fishnets: These never seem to go out of style, and now they come in a wide range of colors and size of netting. Leave the bright colors and super-sized nets to the club kids. You're better off in basic black and a small net. My favorite is Spanx Control Top Fishnets. They're comfortable because the net stops at your upper thigh and is topped with a control-top panty (so no "grid butt").

Sheers: As we said, nude stockings — even the best ones — are OL. "I hate nude hose. I hate colored sheer hose. I much prefer sheer black hose," says Isaac Mizrahi. If you have to wear a sheer stocking, make it black and seamless. It could have a very slimming effect on your overall leg.

Colors: Whether it's opaque tights, fishnets, or

sheers, stick with the classic colors — the fuchsias, yellows, and purples are fun on tween queens. The shades you wear should easily blend (not contrast) with your skirts and shoes to create the illusion of one lean, long line of leg.

Textures: Kooky patterns, flashy prints, thick knits, glittery embellishments, and seams aren't flattering, and they'll call more attention to your legs than you probably want.

Control top: Bring it on! Like good shapewear, control-top panty hose will help create a smooth line under your clothes. Some even eliminate the

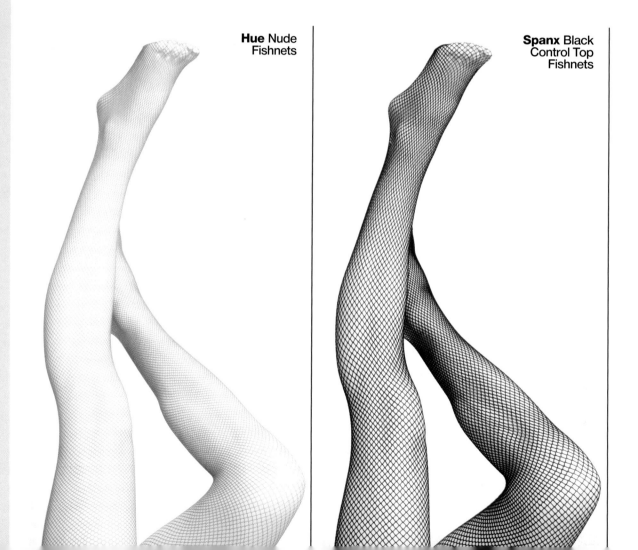

Hue Nude Fishnets

Spanx Black Control Top Fishnets

need for wearing panties, so you don't have to worry about VPL.

Reinforced toes: Okay, there is one thing worse than nude hose — nude hose with reinforced toes! Even if you are wearing closed-toe shoes, you don't want to wear reinforced toes; you never know when you might have to kick off your shoes. And never, *ever* reveal a reinforced toe in an open-toe shoe. It is, without a doubt, the most OL look going.

Socks: The best socks are the ones you don't actually see (and hopefully are so comfortable you don't feel them either). Your pants should never be short enough to show the length of the socks, so be sure your socks extend high enough up your legs so that even when you cross your legs, no skin is revealed. A knee-high trouser sock with a bit of Lycra will feel silky, stay up without binding, and look more like chic opaque tights than a schoolgirl's kneesock. Spanx Two-Timin' Socks hit the right spot and are reversible — black to brown, gray, or navy. Cashmere socks are a cozy indulgence when padding around the house on a cold day, but most are too bulky to wear under boots.

The Newer Way to . . .

Dress Your Legs for Evening When It's Freezing Outside

My biggest legwear challenge is what to do when it's freezing out and I'm all dressed up. I do try to go bare-legged for evening whenever possible, but when heading out the door in subfreezing temperatures, bare legs simply don't work. And since the only thing worse than wearing the wrong stockings is revealing frozen, goose-bumpy legs, it's important to find a chic solution. If you're wearing a light-colored dress, try nude fishnet stockings (instead of nude sheer stockings). With a black dress, you can get away with very sheer black stockings or black fishnets. And if you dare, at least when wearing a short skirt or dress for evening, consider Isaac Mizrahi's Y&H option: opaque black tights with peep-toe pumps. "Why wouldn't you wear black opaques with an evening dress?" Isaac asks. "Who says that's wrong? If you're freezing, it just looks younger and better to me." Go for it!

LET US SPRAY: STOCKING SUBSTITUTES

Leg makeup used to be the messiest thing on the market, and only women with really bad veins to cover up would even bother. But in the past couple of years, leg sprays have hit store shelves.

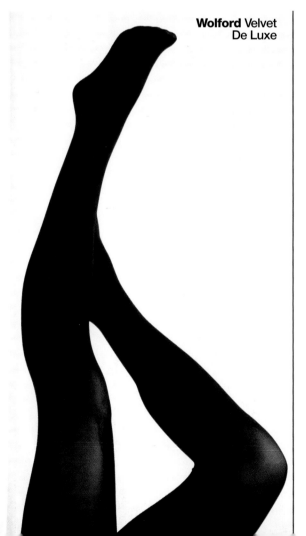

Wolford Velvet De Luxe

Leg sprays cover all your lumps and bumps, instantly giving you the polished look of stockings.

These next-generation stocking substitutes gorgeously cover all your lumps and bumps, instantly giving you the polished look of stockings without getting all over your clothes. I use them every time I go on TV to make my legs look flawless but still bare. Adding at least one of these products to your makeup collection is an absolute Y&H essential. See Brilliant Buys for a few of my favorites.

Michael Kors Leg Shine isn't full coverage or a spray, but rather a sexy, shiny shimmer in a deodorant-like push-up stick. The advantage is that you can apply it on the run, because there's no chance of spillage and no waiting for it to dry.

GETTING YOUR LEGS BARE-ABLE

When you do go stockingless, you need to make sure your legs look good enough to be on display. The appearance of your legs hinges on the appearance of your skin. It needs to be soft, smooth, and hairless, with a little color and no visible veins.

HIGH, MEDIUM, AND LOW MAINTENANCE . . . DEFUZZING YOUR LEGS

Zapping away the hair on your legs requires a different strategy than zapping the hair on your face (see chapter 9). Here's how to get hair-free, whatever your time, money, and comfort level.

HIGH: Laser hair reduction is the gold standard for ridding yourself of unwanted hair, although you have to be either high maintenance or excessively hairy to choose it for an area as large as your legs, because it's time-consuming and expensive. (Lasers are more often used on the face, under arms, and on bikini lines.) Although lasers for hair removal keep improving, it's still difficult to eradicate dark hair on dark skin (and light hair on light skin), because the hair needs to be darker than the skin in order for the laser to differentiate skin from hair. Other reasons why you might not be an appropriate candidate: If you are suntanned or if you are taking certain medications (you need to stop several weeks before it's safe to laser). That's why it's important to go to a health care professional with laser experience, not just someone who took a weekend course in order to be able to rent the laser. "If the technician says, 'Oh, you have a suntan . . . Oh, you're on tetracycline — we'll see you anyway,' that's how you get problems," says laser specialist Terri Levin. The upside to lasers is that after an average of six sessions, you may be done with the hairy leg problem — if not completely, at least for a long time. Average price for the lower leg only is $500 for a one-hour session, which is $3,000 for six sessions.

MEDIUM: Waxing will leave your legs completely bare of hair for a look that's smooth and flawless. It's the method of choice for women who seek perfection — swimsuit models, red-carpet celebs, and, of course, adult entertainment stars. On the downside, it hurts, it's expensive to keep up, it's messy to do yourself, and, worst of all, you have to let about one quarter inch of stubble grow in before you can wax again, so you do have to schedule your "imperfect" time.

LOW: Shaving your legs is the fastest, easiest, and most convenient way to keep them hair-free all the time. All it takes is thirty seconds in the shower every other day. Along with self-tanning (see the next section), it's one of my few beauty routines that fall into the low-maintenance category, and I'm not alone. According to Gillette, 95 percent of American women choose the razor as their leg hair removal method of choice. My favorite razor (sorry, Gillette) is the Schick Intuition, because the blade is attached to a cartridge that automatically releases shaving cream while you shave. I never buy shaving cream anymore, which means no more cans leaving rings in my shower. It's one of those beauty innovations that has you saying, "What took them so long?"

The Newer Way to . . .
Banish Flaky Skin
Legs have to be soft, touchable, and well moisturized to look truly Y&H. Slapping on a moisturizing lotion after your shower is the obvious to-do, but you need the time and patience to let it dry before getting dressed. That's why my savior has been the breakthrough moisturizer you use while still in the shower — Olay In Shower Body Lotion. I slather it all over, rinse, towel off, and I'm done! No waiting required.

HIGH, MEDIUM, AND LOW MAINTENANCE . . . SUNLESS TANNING YOUR LEGS

We all know that spending time in the sun courting a real tan is not an option if you care about (a) getting skin cancer or (b) getting wrinkles, sagging, and age spots. And don't even think of hitting a tanning bed! Why expose yourself to potentially damaging rays — whether they come from the sun or a sunlamp — when you can easily fake a bake? It's so much healthier to get your sun-kissed look with a sunless tanner — and so much better to be in control of your glow and color.

HIGH: If you don't want to get your hands dirty or run the risk of streaks, let a pro apply your tanner for you. At a salon or spa, an aesthetician will exfoliate you from head to toe, then smooth on the tanner. Expect to pay about $75 in New York City (maybe slightly less elsewhere) for this service and to go in once a week or so to keep up the color.

MEDIUM: Get your entire body spritzed with an airbrush or spray-on tan once a week. It's easy and quick — just stand in front of a stream of spray in a private booth. Most franchises that offer the service sell a series of sessions for a slight price break, charging about $45 per session.

LOW: At-home self-tanning is easy to do, and the products available keep getting better — although you do need an hour or so free to walk around the house in a swimsuit while it dries! For the smoothest results, always exfoliate your skin before applying a self-tanner. (If you shave and then exfoliate, it will be painful!) Avoid stained palms by slathering on a silicone hair product first — it'll protect your palms from absorbing the color without interfering with the tanner application. Avoid stained bathroom rugs and towels by standing in the tub or shower while applying. See Brilliant Buys for self-tanners that deliver believable results, have a pleasant smell, and are easy to use.

VAIN? YES! VEINS? NO!

Nothing will ruin the look of your legs faster than a road map of spider veins or, worse yet, bulging (and sometimes painful) varicose veins. As we age, the valves inside our veins can weaken, fill with too much blood, and swell. This OL problem is one that's more easily solved these days — no overnight hospital stay required, and if done correctly, the treatment can last forever. So if you have bothersome, visible veins, see a dermatologist to find out which options are better for you.

I asked Dr. Neil Sadick, whose Sadick Dermatology Center in New York is at the forefront of all things dermatological, to explain.

Sclerotherapy: This method has been around for years, but it is still the gold standard for getting rid of unwanted veins. It involves injecting a solution into the blood vessel, which causes the vessel to collapse and disappear into the body. According to Dr. Sadick, the procedure has been vastly improved. Fewer visits are required, they no longer wrap the legs, the procedure can be done in the doctor's office, and patients are able to go back to work the same day. The cost is $300 to $450 for a basic session.

Laser: Spider veins can be treated with topical lasers that cause them to heat up, coagulate, and close up. The lasers used to treat mild to moderate leg vein problems include the Gemini, Polaris, and Nd: YAG, but they are more successful on lighter than on darker skin. If you go the laser route, two or three sessions ($650 to $850 each) may be required, depending on the veins.

If you don't have unsightly veins yet, can you prevent them from showing up later? Dr. Sadick reports that a study of the causes showed that it's genetic. His plan of attack: "Have parents with good genes, avoid estrogen derivatives as much as possible, don't do high-impact aerobic exercise, and keep a healthy body weight." Well, there's an excuse to avoid high-impact aerobics!

STOCKINGS AND SOCKS

Spanx Control Top Fishnets, style 002, $26; spanx.com or 888-806-7311

Spanx Tight End Reversible Tights with Tummy Control, style 005B, $32; Bloomingdale's; spanx.com

Spanx Topless Trouser Socks, style 010F, $10; Bloomingdale's, 800-232-1854; Spanx, 888-806-7311 or spanx.com

Spanx Two-Timin' Trouser Socks, style 012, $12; Spanx, 888-806-7311 or spanx.com

Wolford's Velvet De Luxe Tights, $49; Wolford boutiques, 800-WOLFORD or wolford.com

LEG CARE

Clarins Smoothing Body Scrub for New Skin, $34; clarins.com

Olay In Shower Body Lotion, $5.69; Target; Drugstore.com

Schick Intuition Plus Shaving Kit for Sensitive Skin, $8.99; drugstores and mass retailers

SELF-TANNERS

Clarins Radiance-Plus Self Tanning Body Lotion, $39; clarins.com

Jergens Natural Glow Daily Moisturizer, $5.99; drugstores and mass retailers

Lancôme Flash Bronzer Instant Colour Self-Tanning Leg Gel with Pure Vitamin E, $28.50; Saks, 877-551-7257; lancome.com

St. Tropez Tinted Self-Tanning Lotion, $37.50; Sephora, 877-737-4672 or sephora.com

LEG COVER

Michael Kors Leg Shine, $32; sephora.com

NYCE Legs, $19.95; nycelegs.com

Sally Hansen Airbrush Legs, $9.95; drugstores and mass retailers

Scott Barnes Body Bling, $48; Victoria's Secret, victoriassecret.com or 800-411-5116; scottbarnes.com

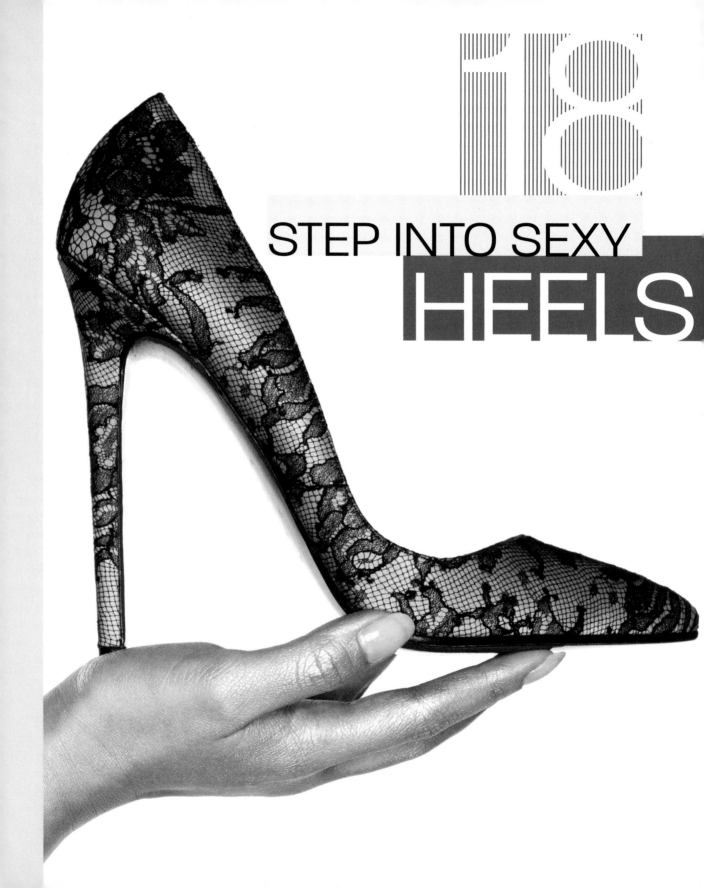

18

STEP INTO SEXY

HEELS

NOTHING AGES YOU LIKE...
UGLY ORTHOPEDIC SHOES... WEARING GYM SNEAKERS OUTSIDE THE GYM... BORING CLASSIC PUMPS... SHOES YOU CAN'T WALK IN... OUT-OF-STYLE SHOES... SENSIBLE SHOES

Most women love shoes. Like handbags and makeup, they are the candy of our wardrobes. But unlike designer handbags, designer shoes do not (yet) cost thousands of dollars, so women can still buy three, four, five, or more pairs each season. And we do! According to NPD Group, which tracks retail purchases, footwear sales to baby boomers (ages 45–64) totaled almost $6.7 billion in 2006, up from about $5.5 billion in 2004.

What has fueled this fire for more and more shoes is that designers have gotten smart. Rather than offering the same old styles or, worse yet, dictating one "in" style of the season, shoe designers are giving us a wealth of choices. With shoe departments packed with so many tantalizing shapes (round toes, square toes, peep toes), heels (stilettos, flats, wedges, platforms), and fabrics (leather, suede, Lucite, velvet, patent leather, metallic), who can resist trying on and buying several new pairs?

I must own a hundred or more pairs of shoes. But as you well know, there's a big difference between how many pairs you own and how many you actually wear. No doubt we all have several pairs of incredibly sexy — and incredibly uncomfortable — shoes that sit in the closet unworn year after year because we like looking at them and can't bear to part with them. I'm here to tell you to stop trying to wear shoes that kill your feet. But wait, before you shudder at the thought of a closet filled with OL-looking comfy shoes, relax. I'm not ready to give up sexy shoes, and I hope you're not either.

Thankfully, you no longer have to sacrifice fit for fashion. The point of this chapter is that you most definitely can (and should!) wear sexy shoes. You just need to be a more discerning shopper and not buy on looks alone. First of all, next time you go to buy shoes, have your feet measured. You may be shocked to learn that you've been wearing the wrong size. (Hmm, no wonder they hurt!) I always thought that shoe size was the one constant in our lives, but that's not true. Each decade, our feet are actually changing slightly in size and shape. So if you haven't had yours measured in decades, chances are you've gone up a size. In fact, according to podiatrist to the stars, my friend Dr. Suzanne Levine, at fifty you should be wearing a full size larger than you wore at twenty.

Make no mistake: I am not suggesting that because your feet got bigger, you have to ensconce them in ugly orthopedic-looking nightmares. The great news is that in the past couple of years, comfy shoes have gotten sexier, and sexy shoes have gotten comfier. Comfort brands such as Aerosoles and Easy Spirit have teamed up with fashion designers to create wearable shoes that look totally Y&H. And fashion brands such as Cole Haan, Stuart Weitzman, and Kate Spade are paying more attention to comfort than ever before. This movement afoot in the shoe industry is good news for all of us and means we'll never again have to choose between looking sexy in shoes and being able to walk in them. What took them so long?

HAPPY FEET: SHOES TO KEEP; SHOES TO TOSS

I'm not going to do what a zillion other books have done before and tell you exactly how many pairs of shoes you need in which styles, shapes, and colors. But I am going to tell you the best and worst styles for women our age.

Keep (or Buy) These

■ **D'Orsay pumps:** A style that's open on the sides (or with an open toe) can be kinder to your feet than one that keeps your feet completely confined. And showing a little skin, or "toe cleavage," is also a very sexy way to look Y&H at any age.

■ **Peep toes:** More Y&H than a boring, basic pump, these shoes with a cutout in the front are still suitable for the office. Just be sure your toes are perfectly polished.

■ **Kitten heels:** These diminutive heels (generally not higher than two inches) have a chic, delicate shape, and their lower height makes them a great wear-all-day option. I even have rubber rain boots with a little kitten heel for navigating wet weather in style.

■ **Sling-backs:** A sexy alternative to the classic pump, the sling-back looks great with skirts or trousers, for daytime or evening. If you have thin heels, to keep the strap from slipping, try the Strappy Strips from Foot Petals, made to hold sling-backs in place. These require bare legs (please don't try to pair stockings with sling-backs or mules), so be sure your heels are pumiced and moisturized.

■ **Stacked heels:** The thicker the heel, the steadier (and more comfortable) you'll be on your feet. This is especially important as the heels get higher: tall and stacked is more stable than a skinny stiletto.

■ **Wedges or platforms:** These stiletto alternatives will give you a little height without the hurt. Because they raise the entire foot (rather than just the heel), your weight is more evenly distributed, and the balls of your feet won't take the same punishment they do with high heels.

■ **Mary Janes:** Straps over the foot add stability to a pair of pumps. A low ankle strap (it should wrap just underneath the ankle) has the added bonus of flattering the foot and elongating the leg.

■ **Fitted, knee-high boots:** These are a perennial favorite, and with good reason. One of your best fall and winter options is to pull on a great pair of brown or black suede boots with matching opaque tights. The look is very slimming, very Y&H, and it covers a multitude of sins (veins, age spots, scars, bruises, you name it).

■ **Ankle boots:** Low heel or high, this is a great look with jeans and pants.

■ **Pointy-toe flats:** We'll talk later in this chapter about why this shape isn't great for your feet (so it shouldn't be one you wear for hours on end), but this style can be a chic alternative to heels, especially if it shows some sexy toe cleavage.

■ **Walking shoes:** I know the very phrase conjures up images of ugly OL shoes, but believe me, there really are cool shoes in this category, from Prada to DKNY. Look for a pair with good support for your arches, good padding in the insoles, and flexible rubber soles. Wear them when you are shopping at the mall, walking through airports, or sightseeing — or at any other time you want to be casually stylish while spending hours on your feet.

Don't give up on heels:
a wardrobe of high and low lets you switch throughout the day

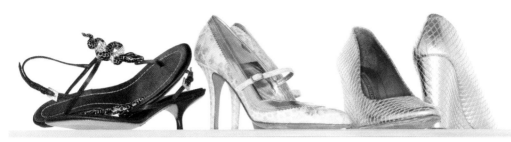

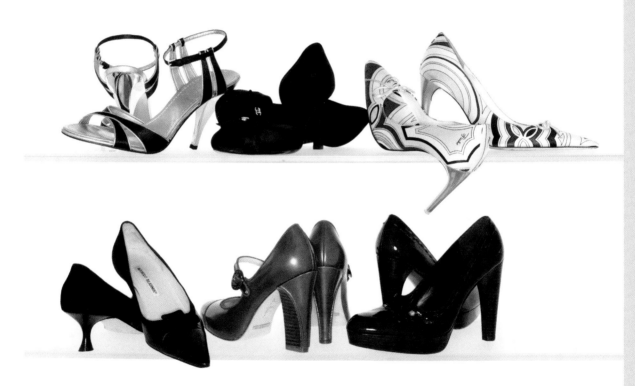

Toss These

■ **Ballet flats:** Flat doesn't necessarily equal comfort. A shoe with absolutely no heel at all gives the foot none of the support it needs. Fake the look with a shoe that has ballet-slipper styling but isn't quite so pancake flat.

■ **Flip-flops:** Save them for the beach or after a pedicure. They look silly in the city, and they offer feet very little cushion for pounding the pavement.

■ **Espadrilles:** A shoe that wraps and ties around the calves is best left to the ballerinas and to taller women. For the rest of us, it just makes our legs look short.

Adopt a Stiletto Strategy

High heels make your legs look good, and they make you feel sexy and youthful. Some women seem to wear them with ease. But if you, like me, have foot problems that make your heels hurt, you need a plan that allows you to enjoy the look without the ache. My strategy is simple: I switch shoes three times (or even more) throughout the day. On my way to work — whether I'm walking, riding in a car, or otherwise commuting — I slip on a pair of stylish walking shoes (the Mary Jane kitten heels from Prada Sport are genius). Once I'm in the office, I change into a pair of comfortable-but-chic work shoes (such as a kitten-heeled sling-back or pump). And if I have a lunch meeting or go out to dinner or an event after work, I break out the sexy stilettos. That way, I'm wearing killer heels only a few hours a day.

■ **Ugg boots:** There's nothing Y&H about wearing the same brand as your thirteen-year-old daughter. Opt for more sophisticated snow wear instead.

■ **High-platform sandals:** According to Dr. Levine, these are your feet's number one worst enemy. Because the straps offer little structure, it's common for the foot to slip off the platform and for the shoe to go one way while the ankle goes the other. Ouch!

■ **Thigh-high boots:** This high-rise style won't do your legs any favors.

HIGH, MEDIUM, AND LOW MAINTENANCE . . . MORE WEARABLE HIGH HEELS

It's not just your imagination — your feet probably do get sore faster now than they did when you were in your twenties. The new pain is due to the loss of your foot's natural padding. Here are three ways to get it back.

HIGH: Injectable padding. Dr. Levine helps women withstand hours in their high heels by injecting Sculptra (poly-L-lactic acid; see chapter 8) into the balls of their feet. The substance is FDA approved for injecting into faces to restore volume (such as plumping up sagging cheeks).

MEDIUM: Custom-made orthotics, which are prescribed by a podiatrist, typically cost $250 and up. Putting these inserts into your shoes helps put your feet into better alignment, which also helps take some of the pressure off the balls of your feet. Another option for making feet more comfortable is to look for shoes with extra padding, such as the Cole Haan line of heels with Nike Air technology. (See the cheat sheet at the end of this chapter for more about these shoes.) These high-tech miracle shoes cost $285 to $350.

LOW: There are several inexpensive options to pad your feet and make your shoes, even high heels, more comfortable. Many podiatrists recommend Insolia, an insert made especially for high heels. Celebs such as Teri Hatcher and Marcia Cross, as well as many high-heeled fashionistas, swear by the various chic padding options made by Foot Petals.

Q&A on Feet

Not everyone has problem feet. If you fall into this category, good for you! For the rest of us, I sat down with Dr. Suzanne Levine to get some explanations for what's happening to our not-as-young-as-they-used-to-be tootsies.

I swear I got a bunion overnight from a bad pair of shoes. Is that really possible?

A bunion is a bony protrusion on the outside of the big toe that develops over years — not from one outing in uncomfortable shoes. They often start to develop in the thirties, and switching away from pointy-toe, super-high heels at that point can prevent them from getting worse. Get your feet measured by a professional, and make sure you're not wearing shoes that are too small. Choose shoes in materials that give, like soft leather and suede. And try inserts — either custom-made orthotics or nonprescription insoles — to help keep feet from rolling inward and putting too much pressure on the forefoot at the base of the big toe. To cushion existing bunions, try over-the-counter moleskin.

How come I used to be able to wear high heels all day without pain, and now my feet ache after just a couple of hours?

By the time you hit your forties, your feet have lost at least some of the fatty cushion that naturally protects the balls of the feet. So with each step — especially in heels — you are putting extra pressure on the feet. It's like wearing out the shock absorbers on your car. You need to look for shoes with more padding to make up for it.

What can I do to get my feet smoother and softer?

The outer layer of skin on the feet thins out and gets drier by the time you hit your fifties. This can cause painful [and ugly!] cracks, especially around your heels. Your best defense is to keep feet exfoli-ated and well moisturized. I use a pumice in the shower every single day. Then afterward, moisturize your feet and slip on a pair of cotton socks for an hour or so. Lotions that contain glycolic acid will speed up the smoothing process by helping skin shed dead layers.

Is years of wearing nail polish to blame for toenails that turn yellow?

The nails naturally get thicker, yellower, and more prone to fungus as you get older. Thickening has a lot to do with circulation (which slows with age), and nail polish and remover can cause some yellowing. If you're concerned about the condition of your toenails, you should see a podiatrist to rule out a fungus as the culprit. Provided your nails are healthy, there's no reason not to wear nail polish, but I do think it's a good idea to remove polish for a day or two in between pedicures.

Do I have to worry about pedicures at the nail salon?

Putting your feet in the hands of a professional pedicurist is a wonderful treat. But it can also be a recipe for disaster if you don't take a few basic precautions. Unsterilized instruments and basins can be the cause of fungal, bacterial, and viral infections. The only way to guarantee a completely safe and sanitary pedicure is to bring your own instruments with you and to clean out the basin with a disinfectant wipe before the pedicurist fills it with water — I actually do this. And never, ever allow anyone but a certified podiatrist to use any sharp instruments to shave away corns and calluses. In fact, if your foot health warrants it, your insurance company might cover the cost of a medical pedicure performed at your podiatrist's office.

Your Shoe-Shopping Checklist

Obviously, what draws us into the shoe department is the lure of fashion's latest styles. But what's going to keep your feet happy are shoes that feel as good as they look. Follow these guidelines when sizing up a new pair.

✔ **The fit:** It seems obvious that you want to buy shoes that fit your feet, but the truth is that most of us don't. Start by getting your feet professionally measured to assess your true size, and if one foot is bigger, try on shoes only in that larger size. Width is also key — a too-narrow shoe will pinch the forefoot together, setting the stage for pain and the development of future foot problems. Test the fit yourself by standing up and pressing down on the tip of the shoe — you should have one thumb's width from the end of the shoe to the start of your big toe.

✔ **The shape**: A square or rounded front that's wide enough to comfortably accommodate all five toes will obviously be the most comfortable. But we all know that a pointier toe looks much, much sexier! So shop for the most wearable pointy toe you can find (sometimes going for a slightly bigger or wider size helps), and if the shoes still hurt your feet, save them for special occasions only.

✔ **The heel:** I'm the first to admit that high heels are fabulous, but most of us can't wear them 24/7 without at least a little pain. According to Dr. Levine, the safest height is a 2- to 2½-inch heel — higher than that, and you run the risk of aching calf muscles and Achilles tendons. Plus, in a 3-inch heel, you're throwing your whole body weight forward and exerting up to seven times the pressure on the ball of your foot. Ideal is a sexy kitten heel, because it's not high or wobbly.

✔ **The material:** As a general rule, the softer, more flexible the shoe, the happier your feet will feel. Look for uppers made from forgiving leather, suede, or a soft fabric such as velvet. The sole of the shoe needs to be able to bend in the forefoot (where your foot naturally bends). If you can't bend the shoe, don't buy it. Padding on the bottom of the shoe is key — even a thin layer of rubber on the sole will increase your comfort level while standing and walking. On the inside of the shoe, it's all about the padding. The more that's in the shoe, the better able you are to walk and stand in it without pain. Test a shoe by pressing your thumb along the ball of the foot area and the arch. If there's enough padding, your thumbprint should spring back.

✔ **The structure:** Although you want a shoe that can bend with your foot, a good shoe can't be flimsy. Look for a shoe that has a solid, structured support for your arch. You also want a little stiffness in the part of the shoe that holds your heel. If it's too flimsy back there, your ankle won't get the support it needs (a frequent culprit in high-heeled, twisted-ankle incidents).

Let's Go Shoe Shopping

Killer shoes don't have to kill. Here are some sole-saving strategies.

- **Shop at midday,** never first thing in the morning. Thanks to gravity, feet tend to swell a bit as the day goes on, so by waiting until afternoon to try on shoes, you will get a clearer picture of how they truly fit.
- **Wear the exact same type of socks,** stockings, or tights that you plan to wear with the shoes when you try them on in the store.
- **Don't just slip on the shoes,** stand up, and admire them in the mirror. You need to take a walk — and not only on the carpeted floor of the shoe store. Shoes feel different on a hard surface, so seek out a wood or tile floor for a true test. (Ask to step out of a carpeted boutique and into the mall.)
- **Don't believe a salesperson** who says you need to "break in" the shoes. It's one of the big lies we fall for because we don't want to pass up a pair of shoes that are so beautiful or on sale — even though they kill our feet.
- **Continue your test-drive** when you bring a new pair of shoes home. Before you wear them outside (once you scuff them, you own them), wear them around the house for a couple of hours to make sure they really are worth keeping.
- **Know the return policy.** Most boutiques will only give you a store credit (which might mean being stuck buying another pair of the same designer's uncomfortable shoes). Whenever possible, buy at a department store, where you can usually get a refund on nonsale shoes.

WHAT THE SHOEMAKER CAN DO

Having a good shoemaker is as important as finding a good tailor. Both can make you look better. A shoemaker who really knows what he or she is doing can turn an uncomfortable pair of shoes into ones you can actually wear, salvage a favorite pair you thought were ready for the trash, or update a style that's not quite this season.

Stretch: Don't buy a shoe that's too tight, but if you find yourself with a pair, a shoemaker may be able to provide some relief. The key is that shoes have to be stretched for a full twenty-four hours. If you go in and leave your shoes to be stretched for just an hour, they will go right back to their former size.

Add rubber soles: Thin, leather-soled shoes are not only uncomfortable to stand and walk in, but they can wear through very quickly. Adding a half sole (it'll cover from just under the arch up to the toes) of rubber will extend the life span and make your feet feel better.

Change heels: You can instantly update the look of an old shoe (or improve the comfort of a pair that are too painful to wear) by having a shoemaker raise or lower the heel; replace a skinny heel with a sturdier, stacked one; or fix a heel that's worn down.

Add padding: To upgrade a shoe's foot bed, insert a cushioned insole or a pad at the heel to prevent slipping (especially important if you have to buy bigger to accommodate one foot that's larger).

Take boots in (or out): A zip-up boot can be adjusted half an inch to an inch so that it hugs your calf as it was meant to.

YOUR CHEAT SHEET TO HEELS THAT DON'T HURT

Of course, not every shoe from every designer is going to be either completely comfortable or a total killer. Even fashion lines such as Prada and Chanel have some shoes with rubber soles or other foot-friendly touches. And stiletto masters Jimmy Choo and Manolo Blahnik offer a variety of heel heights so that you can get their chic style without going sky-high. The recent breakthrough in the marriage of fashion and comfort began when Cole Haan's creative director, Gordon Thompson III, came fresh from a job as corporate vice president of design at Nike and was determined to make Cole Haan's fashionable shoes as comfortable as a pair of Nikes. A collaboration between the two companies resulted in a line of heels called Dress Air, which feature Nike Air padding concealed inside half-inch platforms under the ball of the foot and in the heels. The "fashion meets comfort" concept also has expanded to evening shoes and heels for the bride and bridal party.

Besides Cole Haan, here are a few brands that deserve your attention when you're shopping for non-killer shoes.

Stuart Weitzman: Not all his evening shoes are a walk in the park, but he prides himself on stylish shoes that will last all night long.

Salvatore Ferragamo: This Italian company has been making beautifully comfortable shoes for decades. (Ferragamo himself once custom-made shoes for stars such as Audrey Hepburn and Sophia Loren.) One of the company's claims to fame is that it offers shoes in a full range of widths.

Aerosoles: Next time you're at the mall, walk around and take a look. You can find incredibly comfortable and cute wedges for just $79.

Easy Spirit: In the 1980s, this line's famous ads promised a shoe that "looks like a pump, feels like a sneaker." Well, maybe, but those "sensible" pumps weren't going to make you look Y&H. Now, thanks to a rather short-lived collaboration with Tara Subkoff (co-designer of the ubertrendy Imitation of Christ line), Easy Spirit has gotten

Stiletto masters Jimmy Choo and Manolo Blahnik offer a variety of heel heights so that you can get their chic style without going sky-high.

much more stylish. The company hasn't sacrificed comfort, though, and is using high-tech materials, such as thick Poron padding under the forefoot and gel-like Axidine under the heels.

Naturalizer: They've made a science out of rubber soles, using a super-pliable thermal rubber that conforms to the foot and flexes with your every step.

B R I L L I A N T   B U Y S

SHOES

Foot Petals products, $6.95–$49.95; Foot Petals, footpetals.com

Foot Petals Stiletto Survival Kit, $49.95; footpetals.com

Foot Petals Strut N Style Set, $49.95, footpetals.com

Insolia High Heel Inserts, $8.99–$9.99; insolia.com

FEET

Aquaphor Healing Ointment, $5.99; drugstores and mass retailers

Bliss Softening Sock Salve, $28; Sephora, 877-737-4672 or sephora.com

Bliss Softening Socks, $48; Sephora, 877-737-4672 or sephora.com

DDF Pedi-Cream, $30; Sephora, 877-737-4672 or sephora.com

Lippmann Collection Bootylicious Spa Booties, $48; Bath & Body Works, 800-756-5005 or bathandbodyworks.com

Sally Hansen Foot Mask, $9.99; drugstores and mass retailers

Tweezerman Pedicure Ceramic File, $20; Bath & Body Works, 800-756-5005 or bathandbodyworks.com

Tweezerman Pedicure Kit, $50; Bath & Body Works, 800-756-5005 or bathandbodyworks.com

PEDICURES

Creations by Alan Stuart Pedi Couture pedicure shoes, $17 solids or $20 prints; for info, 800-866-4424 or creationsbyalanstuart.com

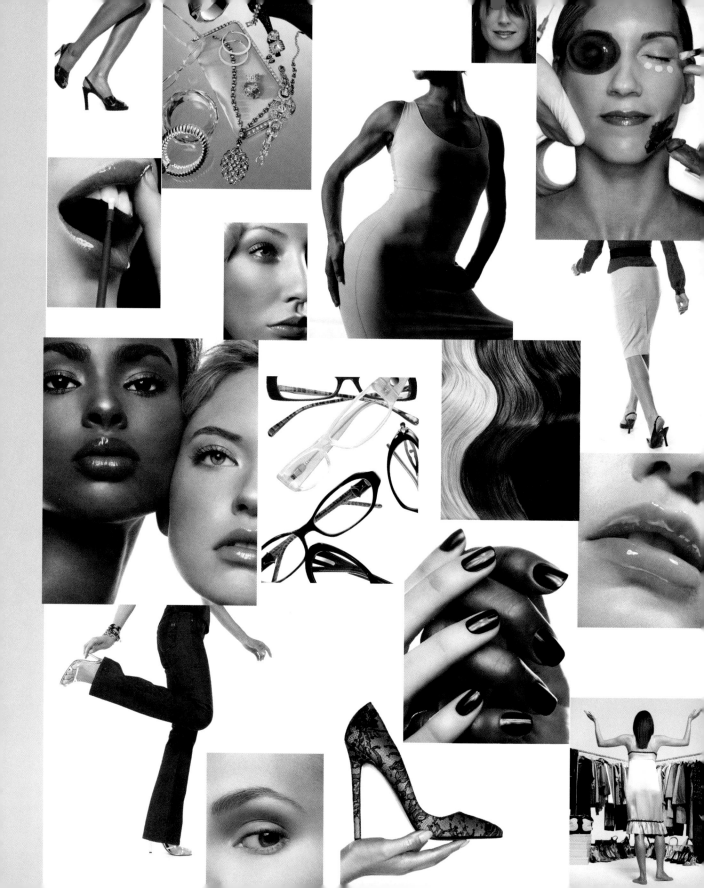

19 PUTTING IT ALL TOGETHER

As I'm writing this, the volume has been turned up on the conversation: What do we do with the rest of our lives? How will we reinvent ourselves in the second act? In her book *Inventing the Rest of Our Lives,* Suzanne Braun Levine writes, "A woman turning 50 in 2005, has a 40 percent chance of living to be 100 . . . so we might as well have as much adventure, satisfaction and life experience as we can." Whether it's finally pursuing passions such as mountain climbing, painting, or politics; going back to school to study art history, French, or a new profession; giving back to the community by joining Habitat for Humanity or traveling to Africa to teach, build infrastructure, or open a school like Oprah, it will be hard to fulfill our dreams on a fixed income. (To say nothing of our Botox bills!) Three out of four of us *do* plan to work beyond age sixty-five, according to a Merrill Lynch study. But can we still work at what we love? That is the question.

Many of us are going to experience age discrimination. In her must-read book *Leap!* Sara Davidson, TV writer and producer, courageously admits that at fifty-seven, she couldn't get anyone in Hollywood to return her calls. One agent explained, "I checked around and I can't sell you to the networks. You don't have an edge," which is Hollywood code for "You're over the hill." Even if no one

at your office says, "Isn't it about time you started thinking about retirement?" you might come to that conclusion yourself when you are no longer in the inner circle, when your boss is a decade or more younger than you, or when it ceases to be fun to go to work every morning.

Pro-age, anti-age — I wish that age wasn't an issue. But in our youth-obsessed culture it is. Until age becomes a nonissue, I don't think it's particularly smart for women to advertise their age. We have always had to work harder and be smarter than our male counterparts — *and look better while doing it.* As Christie Brinkley said in her CoverGirl commercials, "I love being the age I am. I just don't want to look it." No one wants to "look it," because of "age profiling" and the fear of being outed. Why does anyone, besides your doctor, need to know your age anyway? I look forward to the day when asking someone how old he or she is, is considered as inappropriate as asking someone his or her religion or how much she has in the bank. Judge us on our brains, our talent, our spirit, our generosity, our kindness, our warmth, our sense of humor — but not our date of birth, no way! When it comes to employment, judge us on whether we can do the job; that's all that's relevant.

Another reason to make age a nonissue as we rack up birthdays is the love connection. Because women on average outlive men by six or seven years, it's very likely that we will be partnering with younger men. "With the superior longevity of women and their greater likelihood of being left single and healthy, we'll have to get over our collective reluctance to accept the union of an older woman with a younger man," writes boomer authority and futurist Ken Dychtwald in *The Power Years,* in which he predicts that our generation will be winding up, not winding down. "In an AARP survey of singles between ages 40 and 69, one in three women said they had dated a younger man; 14 percent of women in their fifties said they prefer to date men in their forties or younger." And we certainly don't want to look like their mothers!

Have I given you enough reasons why you have to stay Y&H? Keeping current about fashion and beauty, maintaining your looks, tweaking your style seasonally, having a youthful, go-girl attitude — it's the same as diet and exercise. You get on the program (whatever works for you), and you incorporate it into your lifestyle — for the rest of your life. If there is a magic age when you're suddenly allowed to pig out and stop exercising, please tell me! One of my favorite quotes about beauty, "There are no ugly women, only lazy ones," comes from the legendary beauty entrepreneur Helena Rubinstein. She was, to be honest, no beauty, but by attending to her skin, makeup, and fashion, she became wildly successful and transformed herself into one of the most alluring women of her day, charming high society with her impeccable style and delicious wit. I think about her quote whenever I'm tempted to crawl under the covers at night with the day's makeup still clogging my pores.

And from everyone who feels a little guilty about placing so much attention on beauty, I expect to hear the question "What about inner beauty?" My answer: Well, what about it? This is not a *Sophie's Choice* situation. You can have both. "It's

not either/or," says Sara Davidson. "You can focus on developing the inner qualities that make people appealing as they age: charisma, humor, intellectual zest. And you can tend to the outer package, just as you'd refurbish a historical building so it doesn't look run-down or dilapidated." Just don't lay on the paint too thick!

Now, to attend to your outer package, you need to put together your own beauty posse, because no woman can do it alone. You'll do yourself a favor by booking appointments with the best talent in town (that you can afford). On your shopping list, a hairdresser, colorist, and brow pro are the most important. Next, a makeup artist, manicurist, and maybe a facialist and waxer. One weak link, and your look could fizzle. What do I mean? You can spend a lot of money on great hair color and a great cut, but if your brows are too rounded and skinny, you're going to look less than Y&H. Remember that every detail is important. It all counts!

Back in chapter 1, we talked about the democratization of beauty and how every woman can actually "buy pretty." But where? Because a lot of women ask me for recommendations, I decided to put together my own list of the best places to "buy pretty" across the country. After this chapter, you'll find out where to get gorgeous in twenty-one U.S. cities. These are the most coveted addresses and phone numbers, both from my personal BlackBerry and from my network of beauty mavens nationwide. If you're traveling to one of these cities and you need a quick blow-out, you'll know where to book an appointment. If you are still hesitating about treating yourself to the best, keep in mind what Madonna told me when I interviewed her around the time of her first album. Even then, I was taken by the confidence she had in herself. "If you don't believe that you're a star," she said, "nobody else is going to."

The time has come to treat yourself like the star you are. And when you don't look old, no one can tell you that you are too old to do . . . whatever the hell you want!

Your Putting-It-All-Together Top Ten

TEN THINGS YOU CAN DO IN THE NEXT TEN MINUTES TO TAKE OFF TEN YEARS

1. Pick pink for your pout.
2. Arch your brows upward.
3. Cover gray brow hairs with pencil and powder.
4. Slim down your eyeliner.
5. Falsify a few lashes.
6. Don't outline your lips with dark liner.
7. Lighten up on the foundation and powder.
8. Unchain your reading glasses.
9. Lose the suit. Switch up the pieces instead.
10. Slip on heels or high-heeled boots.

TEN THINGS YOU CAN DO FOR LESS THAN $100 TO TAKE OFF TEN YEARS

1. Slim down with shapewear bike shorts.
2. Boost your bust with the right bra.
3. Slough off old skin with a microdermabrasion kit.
4. Switch from powder to cream blush.
5. Cut some bangs.
6. Polish your toes — black, burgundy, whatever.
7. Pick up a hip accessory.
8. Spring for "Body Bling."
9. Whiten your teeth.
10. Have a tailor shorten (and narrow) your skirts.

TEN NEW RULES FOR HOW NOT TO LOOK OLD*

1. Up is better than down (brows, glasses, bust, bum).
2. Soft is better than hard (makeup).
3. Illumination is better than darkness (face, hair).
4. Warm is better than cool (hair color, makeup).
5. Slim is better than heavy (eyeliner, clothing).
6. Moist is better than dry (skin, lips, eyes).
7. Smooth is better than bumpy (eyelids, lips, shapewear).
8. Casual is better than fussy (hair, makeup, clothes).
9. Less is better than more (nails, jeans, legs).
10. And anything is better than nude hose!

*General truths to use where applicable.

STAR STYLES
The Y&H Hall of Fame

Christie Brinkley

Oprah

Sarah Jessica Parker

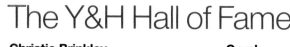

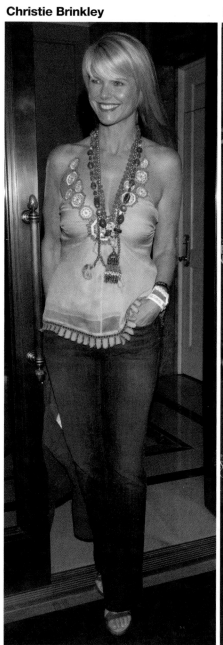

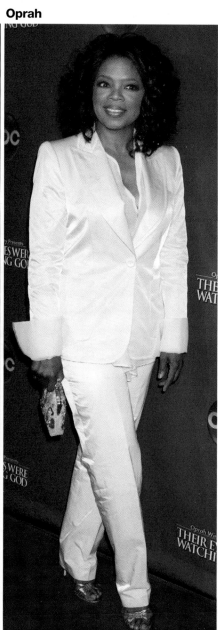

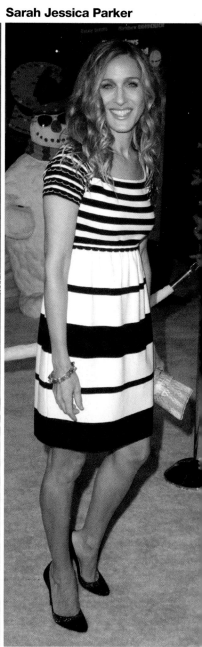

Michelle Pfeiffer   **Demi Moore**   **Madonna**

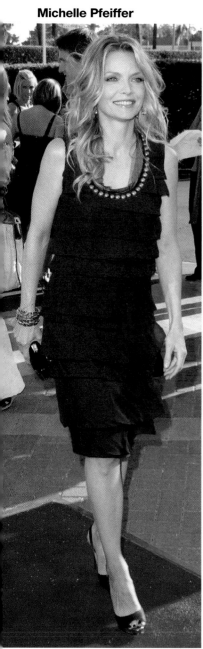
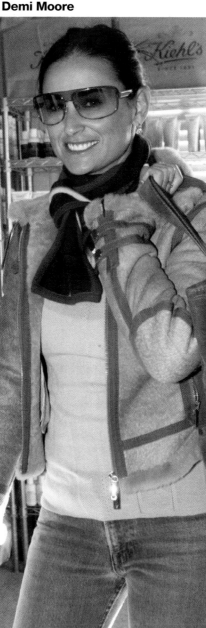
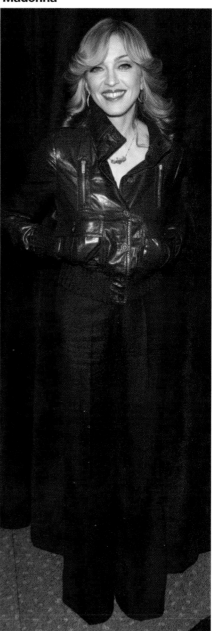

GETTING GORGEOUS CITY BY CITY*

Aspen

Brows

The Cos Bar, 309 S.Galena St., 970-925-6249 or 800-722-8982 (brow styling, $20–$25). Get your brows done and shop at the same time. Long before there was a Sephora, Aspenite Lily Garfield offered all the hard-to-find beauty brands in one stocked shop. Beauty services now include brows and facials. Look for the Cos Bar in eight other U.S. resort towns, including Vail, Carmel, Scottsdale, Santa Fe, and Atlantic City.

Hair

Lather, 600 E. Main St., Suite 1, 970-925-1630 (blow-out, $50 and up; cut, $75; highlights, $125 and up). This "no attitude," full-service salon is where locals and second-home owners go for everything to do with hair.

M Salon, 300 S. Spring St., 970-925-3605 (cut, $85; basic color, $85; highlights, $100 and up). Marcy, the owner, does great color and cuts, and because she's married to the chief of detectives in town, she is pretty much always there.

Nails

Red Spa (Colleen), 205 S. Mill St., 970-925-4648 (regular manicure, $25; French manicure, $30; pedicure, $50).

The Aspen Club, 1450 Ute Ave., 970-925-8900, aspenclub.com (manicure, $35 and up; pedicure,

$60 and up). This is a members-only club, but if you book a spa service, you receive complimentary admission to the health club for the day. Guests at the Hotel Jerome can use the club gratis.

Atlanta

Brows

Aric C. Cosmetics (Aric Castleberry), 3209 Paces Ferry Pl., 404-237-9842 (brow plucking, $25). This makeup artist, salon owner, and founder of his own cosmetics line is an Atlanta favorite for creating the best brow arches for your face.

Azar (Cynthia Craig), 3122 E. Shadowlawn Ave., 404-231-3294 (brow grooming, $25; tinting, $18). Brow perfection with wax.

Facials

Spa Sydell, eight locations, 404-255-7727, spasydell.com (facial, $45–$145). Winner of *Allure*'s Best Facial in Atlanta. Try the antiaging facial with Maka at the Park Place at Perimeter location. A board-certified dermatologist from Soviet Georgia, Maka came to the United States in 2001.

Jurlique Wellness Spa at the Intercontinental, 3315 Peachtree Rd. NE, 404-946-9175 (facial, $100–$145). Aromatherapy facials with the exclusive Australian organic skin care products in a setting that feels like you've jetted out of Buckhead to a resort spa.

Judith of Budapest Skincare Salon (Judith Buran), 550 Pharr Rd., Suite 104, 404-841-1111 (Garden Facial, $87). Judith, who believes that skin care is a necessity, not a luxury, specializes in authentic European-style deep-pore cleansing.

Makeup

Aric C. Cosmetics (Aric Castleberry), 3209 Paces Ferry Pl., 404-237-9842 (makeup application, $45;

*Please note: Prices are subject to change.

makeup lesson, $65). This is the favorite makeup place of Buckhead brides and mothers of the bride, but you don't have to wait for a wedding to get a makeup update or lesson.

Dobél Salon-Spa, 3365 Piedmont Rd., Suite 1250, 404-264-1007 (makeup application, $65 day, $85 night, $250 bridal; makeup lesson, $150). You can easily spend a couple of hours here learning new makeup tricks.

Nails

Jolie the Day Spa (Jonathan Mann), 3619 Piedmont Rd., 404-266-0060 (manicure, $20; pedicure, $40). The extremely meticulous Jonathan includes a twenty-minute foot massage with his pedicures.

Judith of Budapest Skincare Salon (Judith Buran), 550 Pharr Rd., Suite 104, 404-841-1111 (Basic Pedicure, $35; Express Pedicure, $30). It's been called the best pedicure in Atlanta. The hot stone bath, mint scrub, and cucumber cream massage is a true treat for the feet.

Honey Nail Salon & Boutique, 442 East Paces Ferry Rd., 404-816-8340, honeynails.com (pedicure, $40 and up). Honey Nail Salon gets great buzz for its healthful approach to natural nail care. This Buckhead cottage-house spa has a fabulous lounge-like atmosphere, ecofriendly products, and the "honey bee club," where a set of nail tools are stored just for you.

Hair Color

James Madison Salon (Kyle Chandler), The Metropolis, 929 Peachtree St., 404-266-8647 (single process, $70 and up; highlights, $110 and up). Color is an art and Kyle is a master, designing custom highlights that beautifully frame and brighten your face. Especially good with blondes.

Stan Milton Oasis (Jamie Latiolais), 260 Pharr Rd. NE, 404-233-6242 (coloring, $75; partial foil, $120; full foil, $150). CNN's anchorwomen flock to this Buckhead salon for Jamie, who is known for creating smooth, flawless, perfectly colored hair.

Van Michael Salon in Buckhead, 39 West Paces Ferry Rd. NW, 404-237-4664, vanmichael.com (color, $60–$197). This 6,000-square-foot Aveda Concept Salon boasts a big celeb client list and awards for color.

Haircuts and Styling

Carter-Barnes Hair Artisans (Carey Carter), Phipps Plaza, 3500 Peachtree Rd., 404-233-0047 (cut, $110 and up; wash and blow-dry, $35 and up; updo, $85 and up). The salon of choice when designers like Vera Wang, Zac Posen, and Marc Jacobs bring their runway shows to Atlanta.

Bernard Dugaud (Bernard Dugaud), 3090 Roswell Rd., 404-262-9656 (cut, $225 for first appointment, $185 thereafter). Here you can get a meticulous haircut by a sheer perfectionist.

Vis-a-Vis Salon (Todd Puleo), 327 Buckhead Ave., 404-266-3320, visavisthesalon.com (cut, $60–$150). Owned by Van Michael vet Jeffrey McQuithy, it's become one of Atlanta's hottest salons, with a reputation for great customer service, even offering a car wash during your appointment!

James Madison Salon (Aaron), The Metropolis, 929 Peachtree St., 404-266-8647 ($65–$70 with Aaron). *Elle, Marie Claire,* and *Harper's Bazaar* have all named James Madison "the best." Clients include Martha Stewart and other celebs staying at the Four Seasons and Ritz Carlton hotels.

Waxing

Spa Sydell (Jo Walsh), 10593 Old Alabama Connector, Alpharetta, 404-255-7727 (waxing $18–$65). There are eight locations of this well-known Atlanta spa, but at the Alpharetta location Jo Walsh has clients who drive two hours for an appointment with her.

Dobél Salon-Spa (Johnnie Jones), 3365 Piedmont Rd., Suite 1250, 404-264-1007 (waxing, $35 and up).

Boston

Brows and Lashes

LuxLash (Suzanne Cats), 232 Newbury St., 617-587-5274, luxlash.com ($40 and up). Lash and brow extensions at what has been called "the nation's first semipermanent lash and brow spa."

Michaud Cosmedix Studio, 69 Newbury St., Floor 5, 617-262-1607, michaudcosmedix.com. Sarah Pietras for lash extensions ($200 and up) and Julie Michaud for brows ($95 and up). Worth the wait.

Facials

Gretta Cole Copley Place, 10 Huntington Ave., 617-266-6166 (facial, $100). The best facials in Boston, without question.

Makeup

Coco Grace Beauty at the Loft Salon and Day Spa, 98 Addington St., Brookline, 617-277-7797, cocograce.com (makeup by Coco Grace, $150). Coco just may be the city's premier makeup master. She has a celeb following that includes Julianne Moore and Paula Zahn.

Michaud Cosmedix Studio, 69 Newbury St., Floor 5, 617-262-1607, michaudcosmedix.com. Go to Julie Michaud ($200), the fantastic makeup artist who trained at Bumble and Bumble in New York and is credited with bringing lash extensions to Beantown.

Nails and Sunless Tanning

Bella Santé, 38 Newbury St., 617-424-9930, bellasante.com (Bella Bella manicure, $55; spa pedicure, $60; self-tanning, $85).

Gretta Cole Copley Place (Nita Patel), 10 Huntington Ave., 617-266-6166 (pedicure, $50).

Salon Trio (Tatyana), 115 Newbury St., 617-536-0143, salontrioboston.com (pedicure, $50–$60). Salon Trio feels more like a homey apartment than a spa.

Hair

James Joseph Salon, 30 Newbury St., 617-266-7222 (single process, $65 and up; highlights, $120 and up). See colorist Eva Mustafai for dramatic color.

Diego, 143 Newbury St., Floor 2, 617-262-5003 (single process, $60; highlights, $100). Star colorists: Glenn Pereira, David Orlando, and Mark MacNeil.

Salon Mario Russo, 9 Newbury St., 617-424-6676, or 234 Berkeley St., 617-266-4485. For cuts, see Mario himself, who works at both salons ($325 for first appointment, $195 for return visits), and Kent Newton or Gary Croteau at the Berkeley St. location.

Spa

Emerge Spa & Salon, 275 Newbury St., 617-437-0006, emergespasalon.com. A new luxury spa and full-service salon for women and men.

g2o Spa and Salon, 338 Newbury St., 617-262-2220, formerly the Guiliano Day Spa. A full-service salon and spa menu that includes ear candling ($65).

Chicago

Brows

Ayala Maquillage (Diane Ayala), 65 East Oak Street, Floor 3, 312-337-4233, ayalamaquillage .com (first visit, $60). This brow master spends about thirty minutes expertly shaping your natural arches, then filling them in with her own line of mineral makeup powders.

Facials

Spa Space, 161 N. Canal St., 312-466-9585 (facial, $90 and up). Natalie Tessler is a lawyer turned spa owner, and her father is a dermatologist, so her skin-conscious spa serves up medically oriented facials and treatments, including glycolic peels and microdermabrasion. Men, too, will feel comfortable in this cool urban oasis, which also offers body bronzing ($115).

Kiva (Magdalena Mlodojewska), 196 E. Pearson St., 312-840-8120 (facial, $90 and up). Good all-around full-service spa, convenient Water Tower location, open seven days.

Nails

Honey Child Salon and Spa, 735 N. La Salle Dr., 312-573-1300 (crème and honey manicure, $55). Owner Bambi Montgomery has won over Chicagoans with her honey-infused treatments and a salon that oozes with style. Honey Child is also a favorite for mane maintenance and does hair extensions. It's a rare salon that caters to both straight and African American hair.

Hair

Salon Buzz (David Maturo), 1 E. Delaware and 310 W. Superior, 312-943-5454 (partial highlights, $100 and up; full highlights, $140 and up). David colors the Who's Who of the Windy City in this buzzy beauty mecca.

Maxine, 712 N. Rush St., 312-751-1511. For color, see Robert Bennett or Jasen James (single process, $70 and up; highlights, $135 and up). For cuts, creative director Amy Abramite keeps Midwestern hair edgy (cuts, $100 and up). This beautifully designed, full-service salon is one of four Kerastase treatment institutes in the country, the place to go for hairapy on dry and damaged locks. Maxine is also the Chicago flagship for L'Oréal's Professional Haircolor. You can get your nails done here, too (manicure, $25 and up; pedicure, $48 and up).

Charles Ifergan, 106 E. Oak St., 312-642-4484, charlesifergan.com (cut, $85; single process, $65). See Tom or Agnes for cuts, Samantha for color. This top shop also has two suburban locations. If it's a sexy new look you want, see the makeovers on the Web site.

Michael & Michael, 365 W. Chicago Ave., 312-951-0779. Co-owner Michael Jacobson is known for his dry-cutting technique (first visit, $300; follow-ups, $160). Stylist Misako Grimaldi is a rising star. "They cut according to your personal hair needs," says beauty maven Bonnie Kaplan, who books Lisa Buenzow for natural-looking color.

Waxing

Sisters Skin Care and Waxing, 845 N. Michigan Ave., 312-943-8800 or 125C Old Orchard Center, 847-673-1120 (waxing, $45–$75). High-powered women in the Windy City line up early for first-rate waxing by these two Lebanese sisters who are experts at chatting throughout the process so you don't feel the pain.

Sunless Tanning

Spacio, 2706 N. Halsted St., Lincoln Park, 773-244-6500 (bronzing, $55). Your airbrushed tan is applied by a real human being, who can also magically contour so your body looks even more buff.

Dallas

Brows

Eliza's Eyes @ Exhale Spa at the Hotel Palomar (Eliza Petrescu), 5300 E. Mockingbird Ln., 214-370-5800 (initial, $85; follow-up, $65). Eyebrow empress Eliza has taken a tweezer to many famous arches (Oprah, Jennifer Lopez). The studio also offers eyelash tinting, and there is complimentary valet parking at the hotel.

Facials

Renee Rouleau Skin Care Salon, 4025 Preston Rd., Suite 606, Plano, 972-378-6655 or 888-211-7560 (facial, $95–$200). A spa dedicated exclusively to skin care, with a client list that includes Jessica Simpson and Heather Graham.

Nails

ZaSpa (Hotel ZaZa), 2332 Leonard St., 214-550-9492, hotelzaza.com (manicures and pedicures, $85). With an Eastern mystical vibe, ZaSpa is not what you'd expect from a day spa. To make a smooth transition into spa mode, relax in the Big Chill room before entering treatment heaven.

Hair

Richard Hayler at Neiman Marcus (Jennifer Weller for color, Henry Uldall for styling), 400 NorthPark Ctr., 214-891-1252 (single process, $50–$100; highlights, $109–$250). The salon is considered the best in the city, and the majority of clients are blondes. You can get sexy bangs here.

Osgood-O'Neil Salon (JT Osgood for color, Bruce Osgood for hair styling), 3213 Knox St., 214-520-1117, or 6932 Snider Plaza, 214-373-6336 (single process, $65 and up; highlights, $110 and up). When the weather permits, enjoy your services on the Zen-like outdoor patio.

Salon Three Thirty, 2510 Cedar Springs Rd., 214-219-1100, salonthreethirty.com (blow-out, $40–$60). In a salon as sleek and sophisticated as an art gallery, owners Peg Cribari, Yancey Smith, and Eric Culbertson turn out hip, fashion-forward looks.

Toni & Guy, 6121 W. Park Blvd., Plano, 972-202-5550 (cut, $44–$74).

Orange, 2932 Main St., 214-698-2006. The vibe here is young and casual, but fancy Highland Park women come here for the talent. For cuts, see owner and stylist Todd Allen ($95), who worked with Oribe in New York and Miami before moving back to Big D. For highlights, go to Michael Murphy ($250 and up), color director of the Oribe salon in Miami, who has done my hair.

Waxing

Avalon Salon & Spa, 3699 McKinney Ave., Suite 412, 214-969-1901, avalonsalon.com (bikini, $35; extended, $45; Brazilian, $60). This Aveda spa with Asian-inspired decor in the hot West Village area is known for its great Brazilian.

Spa

Spa & Salon at the Four Seasons Resort Las Colinas, 4150 N. MacArthur Blvd., Irving, 972-717-2555. From your hair to your toenails, this full-menu resort will serve you well. Local specialties include a down-home Texas pecan body polish.

Spa at the Crescent Hotel, 400 Crescent Ct., 214-871-3232 (Cowboy Boogie pedicure,

$75; Holiday in San Tropez tanning, $90; facial, $60–$130). It's been called the best spa in the city. Dallas society and celebs (Eva Longoria, Gwyneth Paltrow) come for the ultimate in pampering and luxe. You might have to spend the entire day here!

Denver

Brows

Brows on Upper 15th (Michelle Dinsmore, owner), 2540 15th St., 720-855-3021 (brows, $20). In the Highland 'hood. Michelle has freelanced for Laura Mercier and MAC. You can also get makeup applications, waxing, and facials.

Facials

Spa Universaire (Linda Martinez), 475 W. 12th Ave., 303-629-9070 (European Essential Facial, $80). In this Aveda Concept Spa in the Golden Triangle Arts District, the theme of each room is inspired by a different region.

Makeup

Simply Moore (Michael Moore), 3000 E. 3rd Ave., 303-399-4151 (makeup lesson, $125; $75 for each additional half hour).

Nails

Woodhouse Day Spa, 941 E. 17th Ave., 303-813-8488, denver.woodhousespas.com (manicure, $25–$65). Just entering this historic 1886 home is an experience. Those in the know say that Woodhouse has the best massages and nail services in town.

Hair

Salon Posh (Lisa Stelzig-Nichols), 300 Fillmore St., 303-333-3750 (highlights, $75 and up). Many of Denver's boldface names go here.

Click Salon (Charlie Price), 231 Milwaukee St., 303-399-9469. Award-winning stylist and co-owner of Click, Price has run his fingers over many celebrity heads, from Naomi Campbell to Joan Rivers. He charges $115 for a cut in the Cherry Creek North salon, but for $210 he will come to you.

Three Cutters on Pearl, 485 S. Pearl St., 303-733-0845 (cut, $50). This small neighborhood place does inspired haircutting, making everyone look super-put-together.

Matthew Morris Salon, 277 Broadway, Suite D, 303-715-4673 (cut, $55 and up). Matthew gives Denver women good hair days and will still groom the brows of a chosen few.

Phoebe Hair Apparent (Phoebe Miller), 2609 E. Third Ave., 303-388-8580 (blow-out, $35). Queen Noor has been blown-out by Phoebe.

Rita B Downtown, 1590 Little Raven St., 303-534-4000 (cut, $70).

Waxing

Wax in the City, 1664 Market St., 303-592-2929, waxinthecity.com (bikini, $25 and up). The Mile High City's first nothing-but-waxing salon. Said to be the hottest shop in town, maybe because of its no-tipping policy or the fact that it's open seven days a week.

Zuri Boutique Salon/Spa, 3150 E. Third Ave., 303-377-3377 (Brazilian bikini, $55). As painless as five minutes with no-strip wax can be, right in Cherry Creek.

Sunless Tanning

Gina's Studio (Gina Comminello), 300 Fillmore St., 303-618-4825 (bronzing, $30). Gina also gives makeup lessons. She has worked at Dior and Chanel, and in the words of Lesley Kennedy of the *Rocky Mountain News,* "She's awesome."

Detroit

Brows

Todd's Room (Todd Skog), 239 Pierce St., 248-594-0003 (brow grooming, $30). Expert eyebrow arches (tweeze-only, no wax) and great manicures and pedicures. Plus, the gorgeous apothecary is a veritable beauty playground, carrying hard-to-find lines like Senna (pick up a brow stencil kit!).

Touch Spa (Barbara Deyo), 470 N. Old Woodward Ave., Birmingham, 248-203-0901 (tweeze, $30). Barbara, co-owner and makeup artist, does neat, groomed, subtle brows on her share of local celebs. You can get eyelash extensions here, too.

Facials

Margot European Day Spa (Margot Kohler), 101 Townsend, 248-642-3770 (Signature Facial, $95). With over twenty-five years in business and a wonderful rep, Margot gets the boldface names. Find this elegant spa just across the street from the Townsend.

Om Spa, 22070 Michigan Ave., Dearborn, 313-565-9686, omdayspa.com (facial, $90–$125). "One of the best facials ever," raves one local beauty aficionado. "Om is hip and trendy like a New York spa." For state-of-the-art serenity in hot Dearborn, Om might be the best spa in town.

Makeup

About Face (Robin Manoogian, owner), 402 S. Washington Ave., Royal Oak, 248-399-1330 (makeup application, $95). About Face is where the Clintons have prepped for Motor City events. The salon also does great facials and waxing.

Waxing

Emile Salon and Spa (Kathy Wojkiewicz or Kira Kirzhner), 31409 Southfield Rd., Beverly Hills, 248-642-3315 (bikini, $30 and up).

Hair

Palazzolo, 400 S. Washington Ave., Royal Oak, 248-545-0060 (highlights, $99 and up; styling, $40 and up). This loft-style, full-service salon in downtown Royal Oak is the place for local color and cuts.

Antonino Salon and Spa (Anthony Marsalese), 191 Townsend, Birmingham, 248-258-5990 (haircut, $90 and up). If you're staying at the Townsend, walk across the street for your blow-dry.

Salon 6, 172 W. Maple, Birmingham (with a second location in Royal Oak), 248-282-5600 (haircut, $50 and up; color, $50 and up; highlights, $80 and up). Gorgeous new state-of-the-art space offering more than just hair services. Summerita, formerly of Todd's Room, does eyebrows and makeup.

Houston

Facials

Urban Retreat Skin Care Center (Michael or Maggie), Haddon Square, 1701 S. Shepherd, Suite C, 713-523-1701, urbanretreat.com (facial, $85 and up). Beautifying Houston's social set for over twenty years.

Chrysalis Skin Rejuvenation Center (Sabina Khan), 3910 Kirby Dr., Suite 110, 713-522-2111 (Customized Revitalizing Facial, $85 and up). Houston socialites rave about owner Sabina's nurturing facial.

International Derma Spa, 2015E W. Gray St., 713-520-9898 (facials, $85 and up). Expert facials at a place that still does electrolysis (starting at $25).

Makeup

Façade, 1101-03 Uptown Park Blvd., 713-552-1545 (makeup application, $65 and up; makeup lesson, $125 and up).

Sensia Studio, 1711 Post Oak Blvd., 713-627-0070, sensiastudio.com (makeup application, $50; lash extensions, $250). A Japanese Day Spa that gives master makeup lessons. Also good for facials.

Nails

Nature's Way Day Spa & Salon, 5000 Westheimer, Suite 160, 713-629-9995 (manicure, $31; pedicure, $43 and up). An Aveda Lifestyle salon.

Perfect 10 Nails & Spa, 5161 San Felipe, Suite 140, 713-993-0277 (manicure, $18; pedicure, $35).

Hair

Solution for Hair (Mark Horn), 2428 Brazoria, 713-526-4545 (single process, $90 and up; highlights, $140 and up; blow-dry, $65 and up).

Urban Retreat Day Spa & Salon, 2329 San Felipe Blvd., 713-523-2300 (single process, $55 and up; highlights, $100 and up; haircut, $75 and up; blow-out, $45 and up).

M Salon (Michael Singletary), 3815 Richmond, Suite A, 713-572-3100 (haircut, $90). Michael worked in New York before coming back home.

José Eber and Ceron Salon, 1180-12 Uptown Park Blvd., 713-892-8330, joseeberceron.com (single process, $70–$100; highlights, $120 and up). Ceron is color artistic director, Jaclyn Smith has been to Philippe for styling, and Eber himself (cut, $500) is there every two months.

Petit Chateau Salon, 1737 W. Alabama, 713-522-8877 (haircut, $60 and up; blow-dry, $35). Intimate yet full-service.

Kansas City

Facials

Terry Binns Spa, 121 W. 48th St., Suite E100, The Country Club Plaza, 816-531-2040 (facial, $75). The famous faces of Kansas City know to go to this skin sanctuary in the Sulgrave-Regency condos on the edge of the Plaza, even though it doesn't have a sign. Most popular is the seventy-five-minute facial, which offers deep pore cleansing. Good for manicures and pedicures, too.

Hair

Xiphium (Vilma), 5037 W. 117th St., Leawood, 913-696-1616, xiphium.com (cut, $70; color, $75 and up). *The* place for a color and cut, especially for curly hair. See Vilma, owner of this Aveda Concepts Salon in Town Center Plaza, to be totally up to date in Kansas City.

Naturally Salon & Day Spa, 2450 Grand Ave., 816-471-8138, naturallysalon.com (styling, $29–$63). This full-service Aveda Concept Salon in Crown Center has been around forever and still delivers fresh style. It gets the celebs who are staying downtown. Good with African American hair, too.

Las Vegas

Brows

AMP Salon, The Palms Casino, 4321 W. Flamingo Rd., 702-942-6909 (brow grooming, $40). See brow expert and makeup artist Brandi Llewelyn, who was trained by Hollywood eyebrow guru Anastasia Soare. She also gives makeup lessons (has glammed-up Paris Hilton) for $100.

Facials

Red Rock Medi Spa (B. J. Lang), 5375 S. Fort Apache, Suite 101, 702-597-0304 (facial, $75). Not to be confused with the Red Rock Spa, as this one is not in a hotel.

Nails

Salon & Spa Bellagio, 3600 Las Vegas Blvd. South, 702-693-8080 (pedicure, $135). This salon offers the ultimate pedicure, which includes an aromatherapy oxygen treatment and hot-stone foot massage.

Sunless Tanning

The Spa at Wynn (Amy Dunn), 3131 Las Vegas Blvd. S., 702-770-3900 (airbrush tanning, $95). Dunn gets raves for her handheld-airbrush tanning talents. She can contour your body beautiful and give you abs and biceps you never had . . . that last five to seven days. The spa is open to everyone Monday through Thursday and to hotel guests only on Friday through Sunday.

Hair

AMP Salon, The Palms Casino, 4321 W. Flamingo Rd., 702-942-6909 (cut and blow-dry, $85–$105). Colorist to the stars Michael Boychuck is the go-to guy for local color, with a client list of boldface names: Paris and Nicky Hilton, Kirsten Dunst, Rosanna Arquette. This salon does hair and eyelash extensions, too. You can also find Michael at his new salon at Caesar's, 3570 Las Vegas Blvd. S., 702-731-7791.

The Salon at Wynn (Lilo), 3131 Las Vegas Blvd. S., 702-770-3900 (blow-outs, $100 and up; cuts with Lilo, $175). "This place is what makes Vegas tick," says beauty maven Angela Rich. Master stylist Lilo Raguso, who gives a dry cut that gets raves, was imported by Elaine Wynn from Manhattan's Cornelia Day Salon, and before that he worked alongside John Sahag. A beautiful space where the manicures and pedicures are also winners.

Waxing

Box Body Waxing Boutique, 4750 W. Sahara Ave., Suite 28, 702-893-9993 (Brazilian, $53–$85). The place is so intimate, it's the next best thing to being at home. The staff offers wine to ease the pain—and works wonders on men as well.

Spa

Green Valley Ranch Resort & Spa, 2300 Paseo Verde Pkwy., 702-617-7777 (massage, $130 and up). If you want to get away from the Strip, a quick fifteen minutes away in Henderson you'll find the full beauty treatment—hair, nails, facial, massage—and workouts with yoga and spinning classes.

Los Angeles

Brows and Lashes

Anastasia for Brows (Anastasia Soare), 438 N. Bedford Dr., 310-273-3155 (first visit, $80; follow-up, $65). Anastasia has a T-shirt that says STAR PLUCKER. Hollywood's high (brow) priestess is so in demand by LA's most beautiful (Sharon Stone, Debra Messing, Heidi Klum) that she's branded herself (in select Nordstrom's nationwide).

Senna Cosmetics (Eugenia Weston), 367 N. Camden Dr., 310-274-1028 or 20855 Ventura Blvd., Suite 6, Woodland Hills, 818-347-2528 (brows, $35–$45). Makeup artist Eugenia, the genius behind the Form-A-Brow stencil kit, will tweeze you into an arch angel (without using wax).

The Salon by Maxime (Robyn Cosio), 421 N. Rodeo Dr., Beverly Hills, 310-205-2370 (brows, $50). A twenty-eight-year salon veteran, this bicoastal brow guru wrote the book *(Eyebrows)* on brows. Her famous arches can be seen on Courtney Cox, Susan Sarandon, Gina Gershon, and Nicole Kidman. She believes that "the longer the tails of your brows, the younger you look."

Chroma Makeup Studio (Michael Rey), 9605 S. Santa Monica Blvd., Beverly Hills, 310-274-2155 (brows, $35). This makeup studio is best known for brows and almost painless tweezing. Co-owner and makeup artist Michael once worked for Eugenia Weston, and embraces her tweeze-only, no-wax approach.

Kate Somerville Skin Health Experts, 8428 Melrose Pl., 323-655-7546 (Extended Wear Lashes, $350; Party Lashes, $150). Paris Hilton gets hers here. Extended Wear (individual lashes) lasts six to eight weeks; Party Lashes (three on a strand) two to three weeks.

Facials

Kate Somerville Skin Health Experts (Kate Somerville), 8428 Melrose Pl., 323-655-7546 (Signature Facial, $125). The hottest facialist who gets the flawless faces flawless: Annette Bening, Mariska Hargitay, Kyra Sedgwick, Debra Messing, Sandra Oh, Geena Davis, and Sharon Stone.

Mila Moursi Skin Care Institute and Day Spa, 9255 Sunset Blvd., Suite 102, 310-274-1602, milamoursi.com (Signature Facial, $300). Hollywood's high-maintenance stars buy a series here. Mila manually massages facial muscles to prevent droopiness and loss of shape. Longtime clients: Vanessa Williams, Laurie David, Blythe Danner, and Candice Bergen (for twenty-five years).

The Face Place (Tony Silla), 8701 Santa Monica Blvd., 310-855-1150 (facial, $120). More than thirty years in business and still *the* place to get ready for your close-up. The facials combine extraction and galvanic current and are more about results than pampering. Just ask Michelle Pfeiffer, Rene Russo, or Jewel.

Kinara Spa (Olga Lorencin-Northrup), 656 N. Robertson Blvd., 310-657-9188 (Red Carpet Facial, $150). This very civilized spa, café, and gift shop on trendy Robertson gets as much acclaim for its food as it does for its facials. Halle Berry and Christina Applegate get their glow on here. The café features a three-course "antiaging" menu of tasty spa food by a chef who once tested recipes for Canyon Ranch.

Murad Medical Spa, 2141 Rosencrans Ave., El Segundo, 310-726-0470 (Environmental Shield Facial, $110 for fifty minutes). Near LAX Airport, antiaging expert Dr. Howard Murad's pioneering medi-spa delivers serious skin care that marries medicine and beauty.

Makeup

Byron Williams, 9294 Civic Center Dr., Beverly Hills, 310-276-4470, bybyron.com (makeup application, $200). He makes Rene Russo look even better, and cuts Rachel Zoe's tresses. For a special occasion, you'll be in good hands—for makeup or hair—with the talented Mr. Williams, who also designs clothes. As one admirer puts it, "He can blow and sew!"

Senna Cosmetics (Eugenia Weston), 367 N. Camden Dr., 310-274-1028 (makeup application, $75–$85). She sells her terrific makeup line—including mineral makeup—in all three of her LA boutiques.

Nails

Jessica Nail Clinic, 8627 Sunset Blvd., 310-659-9292, and **Jessica From Sunset**, 124½ N. Larchmont Blvd., 323-461-2979 (manicure, $30; pedicure, $32; house calls, $56 and up). From Nancy Reagan to Princess Diana to Madonna, this famous nail salon boasts an impressive Who's Been Here list. Each appointment starts with a nail analysis. No artificial anything here—just natural, beautiful nails.

Tracey Ross (Ina), 8595 W. Sunset Blvd., 310-854-1996 (manicure and pedicure, $50). One more reason to love LA—you can shop while getting your nails done. Sunset Plaza fashionistas know to book ahead for an appointment with Ina, as she's not there every day. Shopping in this unique boutique is a gossip item waiting to happen, but the fabulous Ms. Ross makes it a paparazzi-free zone by blackening the windows.

L.A. Vie L'Orange, 638½ N. Robertson Blvd., 310-289-2501 ("Always on the Run" pedicure for aching feet, $60). It's a scene but for good reason. The fresh, all-natural products (no smell when you walk in) sound more like lunch than pedicure soaks, and the gourmet snacks don't stop. *O, The Oprah Magazine* calls it LA's number one hand and foot spa.

Hair Color

B2V (Kim Vo), 646 North Doheny Dr., W. Hollywood, 310-777-0345 (highlights, $150 and up). Hairdressers who appear on TV reality shows are not necessarily the best in the biz, but Vo gets kudos from other top colorists (not easy to do). A good blonder, he paints strands at the root to avoid quarter-inch foil misses.

Art Luna Salon (Art Luna or Linda Cho), 2116 Main St., Santa Monica, 310-450-7168 (highlights, $225 and up). Art, a longtime LA hair legend, is as famous for his relaxed tropical patio garden as he is for his California blondes (Reese Witherspoon, Kirsten Dunst). Linda is good with brunettes.

Canale Salon (Michael Canale, owner), 214 N. Canon Dr., Beverly Hills, 310-273-8080 (single process, $110 and up; highlights, $260 and up). If you love Jennifer Aniston's golden-blond color and super-natural highlights, Michael is your guy.

John Frieda Salon (Negin Zand), 8440 Melrose Pl., 323-653-4040 (single process, $150; partial highlights, $350; full highlights, $450). So LA! There's a pool in the courtyard and you can lounge around and sip a chai latte while you wait. Colorist Negin Zand has taken LA's most glamorous from blond to brunette and back again. Among her credits: Cate Blanchett, Kim Basinger, Scarlett Johansson, Nicole Kidman, and Penelope Cruz.

Neil George Salon, 9320 Civic Center Dr., Beverly Hills, 310-275-2808 (color, $100 and up; highlights, $175 and up). When British hairdressers Amanda George and Neil Weisberg opened in 2005, Neil said, "We wanted to create a strong team." Color heavyweights Lorri Goddard Clark and Tracey Cunningham came from John Frieda, and Justin Anderson from Art Luna. Clarke has colored Madonna and Cameron Diaz. Tracey Cunningham has done Renée Zellweger, Rebecca Romijn, and Molly Sims. Justin Anderson, aficionados say, "does the absolute best California beach blond."

Haircuts and Styling

Chris McMillan (Chris McMillan or Sally Hershberger), 8944 Burton Way, 310-285-0088 (cut with Chris, $600; cut with Sally, $800). What you may not know about Jennifer Aniston's hairdresser friend is how much he's done to loosen up red-carpet do's with long, laid-back, surfer-girl layers.

Sally, bicoastal rock star of the hair world, does super-cool cuts that erase ten years. One beauty maven calls stylist Kristof Ball (blow-out, $85), "the best at blow-drying on the planet."

Allen Edwards Salon & Spa, locations in Brentwood, Woodland Hills, and Studio City, 818-763-4005 (cut, $65 and up). With three full-service salons in town, the mane man behind Farrah's iconic seventies do remains one the most well-known names in LA hair.

Privé, 7373 Beverly Blvd., 323-931-5559 (cut, $100 and up; blow-dry, $65 and up). Owner Laurent Dufourg, who has bobbed his share of Hollywood power players, splits his time between here and his salon in New York's Soho Grand. Jennifer Negrette, who worked in the trenches with José Eber for ten years, does a great blow-dry.

Frédéric Fekkai, 8457 Melrose Ave., 323-655-7800, or 440 N. Rodeo Dr., 310-777-8700 (blow-out, $75). The newer Melrose space is more intimate than the Beverly Hills mecca, with an outdoor terrace designed for multitasking manis, pedis, and lunch.

Sunless Tanning

Ona Spa, 7373 Beverly Blvd., 323-931-4442 (full-body spray tan, $65; Tan on Wheels, $145 and up). You can go to Ona (above the Privé salon), or Ona can mist you in the privacy of your own shower.

Nava Hadad Skin Care, 931 N. La Cienega, 310-360-9040 (spray tan, $65). Beauty maven Angela Rich calls Nava's "one of the best spray tans in the city."

Chocolate Sun, 204 Bicknell Ave., 310-450-3075 (spray tan, $55). A chem-free spray tan steeped in antioxidants and SPF 30, airbrushed with painterly perfection. No wonder it's a hit with the Santa Monica crowd.

Waxing

Nance Mitchell Beverly Hills, 330 N. LaPeer Dr., 310-276-2722 (bikini wax, $45–$65). When it comes to very personal grooming, Nance has seen (and done) it all—from Brazilians to stylized logos!

Four Seasons Spa, 300 S. Doheny Dr., 310-786-2229 (bikini wax, $50). For waxing (or manicures and pedicures), you can't go wrong here.

Miami

Brows

Rikrak Salon (Leticia Collazo), 1428 Brickell Ave., 305-371-5577 (brows, $50 for first visit, $40 thereafter). Leticia once traveled the world working with Oribe, and now that she's back in Miami, local glamazons (Jennifer Lopez among them) take advantage of Leticia's awesome tweezing talents at this much-buzzed-about, all white, 5,500-square-foot full-service salon. With its own trendy in-house boutique and European coffee bar, it often plays host to parties with guest lists that include Beyoncé.

Laura Di Niro, 305-LUCKY-ME or 305-582-5963, thebrowshoppe.com. (brows, $40 and up). Laura calls herself "The Brow Queen" and buzzes about various parts of Miami, depending on the day. To catch up with her, it's best to check her Web site so you can make an appointment in your neck of the woods.

Some Like It Hot, Browne's Beauty Lounge, 841 Lincoln Rd., 305-538-7544 (brows, $19). Good for manicures ($17) and pedicures ($33), too.

Facials

Millie Lopez at Facemaker Spa Lounge on South Beach, 1307 Eighteenth St., 305-861-1255 (facial, $85 and up). Miami beauties flock to Millie, who worked for dermatologist Diane Walder for fifteen years. Even women with acne-prone skin leave glowing and hydrated.

Elemis Spa, 330 San Lorenzo Ave., 305-774-7171 (Pro-Collagen Japanese Silk Booster, $125). Elemis recently opened in the Loews Hotel, too.

Makeup

Robert Steven Muñoz, 305-205-8733 (makeup application, $150 and up). If you have an event to attend, this is the guy to book.

Nails

Agua at Delano, 1685 Collins Ave., 305-674-6100 (manicure, $40; pedicure, $60). Even the humble manicure gets Agua's full-on, excellent spa service.

Hand & Foot Company, 5792 Sunset Dr., 305-668-0504, thehandandfootcompany.com (manicure, $17–$50; pedicure, $30–$80; Rescue Me Pedicure, $122). Owner Antonia Moforis consistently gets high grades from all those who love baby-soft feet, including Madonna and Jada Pinkett Smith. Her creative concoctions are mixed with natural ingredients — coconut cream, almond-milk beeswax, carrot seed oil — that seem good enough to eat.

Sunless Tanning

Le Spa Lancôme, 150 Eighth St., 305-674-6744 (self-tanning, $50). For a longer-lasting faux tan, go here before you hit the beach. The spa uses only Lancôme products, including the famous Flash Bronzer.

Tan2U, 786-554-5932 (self-tanning, $75 and up). Have Gigi Zunjic and her streak-free airbrush machine come to you! It's said that some celebs keep her on speed dial, but she doesn't spray and tell.

Hair Color

Scott Alan Hair Studio, 20504 West Dixie Highway, 305-931-0500 (single process, $50 and up; highlights, $125 and up). Women in Miami love Scott Alan right now. Also, Ilana Gorin does a great, reasonably priced cut (starting at $50) and blow-out ($35 and up) with an amazing (no charge) scalp massage.

Pipino Salon South Beach, 1901 Collins Ave., 305-534-5554 (single process, $90). This talented colorist keeps demanding divas like Mary J. Blige and Tara Reid coming back for more.

Haircuts

Oribe Salon, 1627 Euclid Ave., 305-538-8006 ($100 for a cut by the staff, $400 for one by Oribe). Still the hottest hair guy with the hottest salon in Miami. If Oribe is out tending to one of his celebrity clients (Jennifer Lopez, Penelope Cruz), see one of his staff members. "Oribe sets a really high bar. If you're not good, you're out," says one local hair pro. If it's extensions, clippings, or falls you're after, this is the place.

Pipino South Beach (Ric Pipino), at Shore Club Hotel, 1901 Collins Ave., 305-695-3296 (cut, $300). Celebrity stylist Ric Pipino, the ex of Heidi Klum, has tons of model and celeb clients (Nicky Hilton, Molly Sims, Naomi Campbell) who see him here or at his Manhattan salon. You've seen his fashion work (Victoria's Secret, Ralph Lauren, Donna Karan) and maybe even Ric himself in the movie *Zoolander* (he played Ben Stiller's stylist).

Hair Styling

Jonny Levy, 305-527-8862 (styling, $100 for a house call). With the heat and humidity in this city of glam nightlife, you always need your hair freshly blown. After twenty years of hairstyling in Manhattan, Jonny Levy and his blowdryer are now permanent fixtures on the Miami scene, and the good news is that he will come to you for a special event or even just for a night out. Sheryl Crow, Natasha

Richardson, Diane von Furstenberg, and I have all relied on the dependable talents of Jonny.

Waxing

Agua Bathhouse Spa at the Delano Hotel (Aida Torres), 1685 Collins Ave., 305-674-6100 (bikini wax, $45). Extreme luxury at this rooftop setting: everything is cushy, white, and billowy.

J. Sisters International, 669 Lincoln Lane N., 305-672-7142 (Brazilian bikini wax, $55). The seven Brazilian sisters are practically an institution in Miami. They also have a salon in Manhattan.

Delia Bernardino, 701 Brickell Key Blvd., 305-582-2517 (bikini wax, $25 and up). Delia counts Madonna among her celebrity clients.

Minneapolis

Brows and Lashes

Extrados, 3100 W. 50th Street, 612-920-0227, extrados.com (brow grooming, $30 and up; brow tinting, $25 and up; eyelash perming, $65 and up; eyelash tinting, $35 and up; eyelash extensions, $150 for a partial set and $300 for a full set). Leah Simon-Clarke, the founder and owner of this chic brow boutique, is *the* brow expert of the Twin Cities. She recently opened a second location in Wayzata and a third in Minneapolis.

Hair Color

Moxie Uptown Hair Salon & Art Gallery, 2649 South Lyndale Ave. S., 612-813-0330 (single process, $50–$75; highlights, $50–$100 and up). Owner Stephen Adams is known for creativity and innovation. Located in the heart of artsy Lyn-Lake, this understated salon caters to an eclectic crowd and attracts up-and-coming stylists.

Haircuts and Styling

Jon English Hairspa Uptown, 1439 West Lake St., 612-824-2474 ($135 for a cut by Linda English; $35 and up with staff; foil, $104 and up; updo, $164; blow-out, $30–$95). Jon, the veteran, no longer cuts, but his wife has taken over. This is the first stop for celebs like Mikhail Baryshnikov, Janet Jackson, and Daryl Hannah.

Denny Kemp Salon-Spa (Denny Kemp), 322 Hennepin Ave. E., 612-676-0300 (cut and blow-out with Denny, $130; with staff, $35–$70). This fresh, edgy alternative in northeast Minneapolis has its share of hush-hush clients. Denny believes that hair color should be casual to suit Minneapolis's active outdoor lifestyle.

Juut Salonspa, Gaviidae Common (Woody Theis), 651 Nicollet Mall, 612-332-3512 (style, $120 with Woody). Woody, a master stylist for Aveda, is one of the best. She has a lot of notable clients in town and is always doing hair backstage at the New York fashion shows.

Root Salon, 499 Selby Ave., St. Paul; 651-222-0200, rootsalons.com (cut, $25–$100). Owner Jim Koktavy is great for makeovers, and he starts every appointment with a beauty consultation. Root also specializes in extensions and special-occasion hair.

Brian Graham Salon, 220 Washington Ave. N., 612-333-3091, briangrahamsalon.com (cut, $35 and up). One of the few chic salons in the Twin Cities that is totally adept at working with African American hair, says Allison Kaplan of the Pioneer Press.

Nashville

Brows

Private Edition Grace's Plaza, 4009 Hillsboro Pike, 615-292-8606 (brows, $15 and up).
The Beauty Lab at Jamie (Lisa Galbraith), 4317 Harding Rd., 615-292-7055 (brow waxing, $25). The Beauty Lab is inside Nashville's best fashion experience, the designer boutique Jamie.

Facials

The Beauty Lab at Jamie (Lisa Galbraith), 4317 Harding Rd., 615-292-7055 (Natura Bisse Diamond Facial, $150). This facial is so popular that even Faith Hill partakes.
Private Edition Grace's Plaza (Kay Winslette), 4009 Hillsboro Pike, 615-292-8606 (Premiere Facial, $70). Private Edition does every kind of waxing, too.
Tiba de Nuhad Khoury Spa, The Mall at Green Hills, 2126 Abbott Martin Rd., 800-964-6868 (facials, $90–$195). LeAnn Rimes and Martina McBride are regulars.

Makeup

Private Edition, Grace's Plaza, 4009 Hillsboro Pike, 615-292-8606. With prestige brands like Laura Mercier and Crème de la Mer, it's not hard to spend $50 here, and when you do, the makeup session is free. The first of beauty entrepreneur Linda Roberts's four Nashville cosmetic emporiums, it's chockablock with the best in beauty. You might run into Ashley Judd or Faith Hill here.
Therapy Systems Store, The Mall at Green Hills, 2126 Abbott Martin Road, 615-292-0202. Therapy Systems offers a menu of facial treatments—including a complimentary Express Facial, glycolic peel, or microdermabrasion—with a $50 purchase from its famous skin care line. No appointments necessary for a five-minute brow fix from Mandi.

Woo Skin Care & Cosmetics, 2154 Bandywood Dr., 615-383-2170. Woo Caroland's beauty boutique sells Chantecaille, Dermalogica, and Fekkai, and there are always in-store events with visiting makeup artists.

Nails

Signature Nails Spa, 3900 Hillsboro Pike, 615-292-6838 (manicure, $15; pedicure, $28). This beauty haven across from the Green Hills Mall may be the best place to get nailed in Nashville. You're served white wine or a complimentary drink while watching a flat-screen TV and getting pedicured with OPI or Essie.

Hair

Element Salon, 2218 Bandywood Dr., 615-727-8484 (haircut, $75 and up). Where the discriminating women of Belle Meade get gorgeous. Stylists Jody Scissom and Kevin Moser, who once cut hair inside Jamie boutique, offer their A-list clients the luxury of a full-service salon, including pampered nail care.
Michealle Vanderpool Salon, 2916 West End Ave., 615-414-3956 (haircut, $65–$250 and up). Book Michealle herself for color, a haircut (which may take two hours), or makeup. She's worked all over in TV and movies, and now this star colorist and makeup artist has opened her own shop.
Rodney Mitchell Salon, 1816 21st Ave. S., 615-460-7002, or The Factory, 230 Franklin Rd., Franklin, 615-599-0559 (haircut, $50–$90). Rodney is a fixture in town, and throughout his career he's had his hands in some famous heads of hair, including those of Shania Twain, Martina McBride, and Faith Hill.

Spa

Relache Spa at the Gaylord Opryland Hotel, 2800 Opryland Dr., 866-972-6779. If you're staying here and want to indulge, the executive spa package includes a pedicure, massage, facial, and hair treatment for $285.

New York City

Brows and Lashes

Robert Sweet William at Barneys New York, 660 Madison Ave., 212-833-2606 (brows, $65). The *New York Times* named Barneys's Brow Man the best in the country. Robert says, "Plucking is for chickens." Instead, he pulls out a magnifying glass and tweezes with exacting precision, creating classy, ladylike brows that then get filled in with powder: a fifteen-minute brow lift.

Christine Chin Spa (Christine Chin), 79 Rivington, 212-353-0503, christinechin.com (brows, $52). Tweezers, scissors, wax . . . Christine utilizes all three on her pretty, devoted following. Can Hilary Swank, Penelope Cruz, and Kate Moss be wrong? Christine is also known for her facials.

RamySpa, 39 E. 3lst St., 212-684-9500, ramy .com (brow grooming with Ramy, $75; with staff, $50). Ramy Gafni, a grooming guru who started out doing brows in the Brad Johns salon, now has his own salon, his own makeup line (Ramy Beauty Therapy), and has even given Britney Spears a makeover.

Pierre Michel, 131 E. 57th St., 212-755-9500 (lash extensions with Monica Crouch, $300). In two hours, Monica glues fifty to sixty lashes onto each lid, resulting in flirty, thick, beautiful lashes—no need to wear mascara for two months. Monica was one of the first in New York to do this, and she remains at the top of the list.

Facials

Ajune, 1294 Third Ave. at 74th St., 212-628-0044 (Mini-Glow facial, $65; Ultimate Ajune Glow, $225). Their Ultimate Ajune Glow restores radiance with the help of a glycolic peel and an LED light non-thermal laser to boost collagen. Ajune, an impressive medi-spa created by a plastic surgeon, offers the latest in high-tech antiaging facials yet doesn't feel hard-sell or intimidating. An oasis of serenity on the Upper East Side.

Jo Malone (Kristen Kammeraad), Flatiron Building, 949 Broadway, 212-673-2220 (facial, $180). No popping or poking, but lymphatic drainage and total pampering using Jo Malone's delicious products.

Paul Labrecque Salon and Spa (Regina Viotto), 160 Columbus Ave., 212-988-7816, or 171 E. 65th St., 212-595-0099 (facial, $110). Regina is always up on the latest skin care, and brings it into the salon where you can buy hard-to-find beauty lines such as Clé de Peau and Santa Maria Novella.

Salon De Shyou, 120 Thompson St., 212-334-4353 (facial with Shyou Hung, $155). Shyou Hung is a master who leaves skin looking better than it ever has before. I originally met her at the Brad Johns Salon before she opened up her own SoHo salon.

Tracie Martyn, 59 Fifth Ave., Suite 1, 212-206-9333 (Resculpting Facial with Tracie, $460; with staff, $325). Tracie's facial—combining microdermabrasion, electronic muscle stimulation, and oxygen mist—is among the priciest in the city, but her results appear to be age-defying. On her client list: Madonna, Susan Sarandon, Linda Evangelista, and Diane von Furstenberg.

Yasmine D'Jerradine, 30 E. 60th St., 212-588-1771; 382 Montauk Hwy., Wainscott, Long Island, 631-537-7300 (Remodeling Facial, $195). Her Upper East Side salon is Moroccan-inspired; her space at the Sage Spa in the Hamptons has an earthier, natural feel. The signature Remodeling Facial uses electrocurrent to sculpt New Yorkers glam.

Naturopathica, Red Horse Plaza, 74 Montauk Hwy., East Hampton, 631-329-2525 (Pure Results Facial, $110). The year-round best place for facials (and massages) in the Hamptons, Barbara Close's modern apothecary embraces you with the scent of lavender and takes your stress levels down a notch as soon as you walk in. There's an integrity here about pure products and stellar service that you just don't find often.

Cornelia Day Resort (Joanna or Anna), 663 Fifth Ave., 8th floor, 212-871-3050 (facials, $175 and up). Celebrated facialist Cornelia Zicu has left the building, but her namesake day resort remains the most opulent beauty sanctuary in Manhattan. It's 22,000 square feet, eight stories above Fifth Avenue, and facials here are a two-person operation (one to attend to hands and feet). Butlers in the Relaxation Library serve fruit and champagne, and the rooftop in summer is open for massages, sunbathing, European baths, and dining. Cornelia set out to redefine the luxury day spa—and spared no expense. The place to spend the better part of a day with friends, celebrating a special occasion.

Makeup

Julie Tussey at Warren Tricomi, The Plaza, Fifth Avenue and 59th St., 212-262-8899 (makeup, $101). This Laura Mercier–trained makeup pro is a find. Call for an appointment because Julie isn't there every day.

Kimara Ahnert Salon, 1113 Madison Ave., 212-452-4252 (makeup with Kimara, $100; lesson, $200; lashes, half set, $25 and up). Before a big event, Upper East Siders book appointments with Kimara, in her jewel box of a shop.

Jason Ascher at Barneys New York, 660 Madison Ave., 212-833-2782 (makeup application, free). When you're ready to turn it up a notch and embrace your inner diva, Jason promises to do it for you with as few steps as possible. No charge for a makeup application because you undoubtedly wind up buying whatever magical potions he uses.

Maribeth Madron, 917-805-6225, maribeth madron.com (makeup application, $250 and up; eyebrow, $75). Maribeth spent ten years working as a Laura Mercier international makeup artist and trainer. Now this experienced artist and eyebrow pro will come to you. She's also available for bridal parties.

Nails

Dashing Diva, 41 E. 8th St., 212-673-9000; 590 Columbus Ave., 212-877-9052; or 1341 Second Ave., 212-570-0770 (basic manicure, $15; All-Out Diva Manicure, $38). It's fun, pink, clean, and not expensive. The perfect place for a manicure party or some mother-daughter bonding.

J. Sisters International (Jonice), 35 W. 57th St., 212-750-2485 (manicure, $45; pedicure, $65). These seven sisters from a beach town near Rio pride themselves on serious nail care. This is not a fast-service place but a meticulous one, where manicures can take an hour and pedicures up to two hours.

Rescue Beauty Lounge, 8 Centre Market Pl., 212-431-0449; or 34 Gansevoort St., 212-206-6409 (manicures, $28 and up). Ji Baek is a self-described "germ-o-phobe" who prides herself on reinventing the typical nail salon. Hers conform to hospital-standard cleanliness and do not reek of acetone. No wonder it's supermodel central.

Warren Tricomi, The Plaza, Fifth Avenue and 59th St., 212-262-8899 (manicure, $31 and up; pedicure, $66 and up). In the new salon at the Plaza, the vibe is retro Hollywood glamour. Think black-and-white photos of Marilyn Monroe and Frank Sinatra.

Ajune Spa, 1294 Third Ave. at 74th St., 212-628-0044 (Clinical Manicure, $50). An antiaging manicure that includes microdermabrasion and LED light waves.

Jin Soon Natural Hand and Foot Spa, 421 East 73rd St., 23 Jones St., or 56 E. 4th St., 212-473-2047 (milk-and-honey pedicure, $50; Spirit of the Beehive Manicure with Paraffin Wrap, $35). Jin Soon Choi, who does a lot of editorial magazine shoots, delivers big results in her three small spaces.

Institute Beaute, 885 Park Ave., 212-535-0229 (Foot Facial, $225). When your feet need serious attention, a nurse at Dr. Suzanne M. Levine's medi-spa will give them a facial, which includes assessing cosmetic foot problems, callus removal, a scrub, mint mask, alpha-beta peals, and nail bleaching.

Sunless Tanning

Clarins Skin Spa (Ingrid Renouard), 1061 Madison Ave. at 80th Street; 212-734-6100 (self-tanning, $125 for one hour). All spa experiences should leave you feeling so renewed. Yes, you can buy the same tube of self-tan milk, but the exfoliation here is so rigorous—and is done with hands, not mitts, as the staff believes in the power of touch. You feel as if you're getting two treatments in one: a massage plus a natural-looking tan that appears two hours later.

Paul Labrecque Salon & Spa, 160 Columbus Ave., 212-988-7816, or 171 E. 65th St., 212-595-0099 (Air Bronze, $95; with exfoliation, $140). The Air Bronze is available at both locations, but on different days, so call ahead.

Elizabeth Arden Red Door Spa, 691 Fifth Ave., 212-546-0200 (St. Tropez Express Body Bronzer, $95; St. Tropez Body Bronzer, $145). The spa uses the same St. Tropez products here as in the other Red Door salons, but prices are $5 higher at the flagship.

Hair Color

Elizabeth Arden Red Door Spa (Brad Johns), 691 Fifth Ave., 212-546-0200 (single process, $200; highlights, $400). Mei is excellent, but it's all about Brad here. Manhattan's power blondes travel from salon to salon wherever this artiste, who has trained many of the city's best colorists, sets up shop. One of his devotees, Lois Johnson of *More* magazine, recently remarked, "We will never allow Brad to retire, ever."

Oscar Blandi, 746 Madison Ave., Floor 2, between 64th and 65th sts., 212-988-9404 (single process, $85–$150, highlights, $175 and up). Beauty PR maven Maury Rogoff, who goes to Frank Friscioni, raves: "Love him, the I-get-stopped-in-the-streets-by-strangers kind of love."

Rita Hazan Salon (Rita Hazan), 720 Fifth Ave. at 56th St., Floor 11, 212-586-4343 (with Rita, single process, $225; highlights, $550). Jennifer Lopez, Eva Longoria, and Brooke Shields are just a few of Rita's fans. She is especially good with rich, sexy brunettes.

Serge Normant at John Frieda Salon (Renee Patronik), 30 E. 76th St., 212-879-1831 (single process, $160; a half head of highlights, $300 and up). Renee, who works only at the uptown location, puts the *wow* in brown.

Haircuts and Styling

Elizabeth Arden Red Door Spa (Chris Cusano), 691 Fifth Ave., 212-546-0200 (cut, blowdry, styling, $175). It's Chris and only Chris here. Chris and Brad Johns have been a cut-and-color duo for years. He cut all three models in this book—and knows from sexy bangs.

Devachan Salon, 560 Broadway, 212-274-8686 (cut, $75–$250). Co-owner Lorraine Massey has created a popular haven for curly girls. Devachan does color, too.

Garren New York Salon, Sherry Netherland Hotel, 781 Fifth Ave., Mezzanine, 212-841-9400 (cut with Garren, $700; with other stylists, $100–$225). For dramatic hair reinvention, it's hard to beat Garren, who has styled the hair of many an icon: Oprah, Madonna, Nicole Kidman, Kate Moss, Angelina Jolie . . .

Orlo Salon (Orlando Pita), 34 Gansevoort St., 212-242-3266 (cut with Orlando, $800; with other stylists, $225 and up). This minimalist four-seat salon in the meatpacking district is home of the $800 signature razor haircut by hair god Orlando, who has cut Madonna, Naomi Campbell, Gwyneth Paltrow, and countless models for magazine covers and runway shows. A haircut by Orlando may be the highest in the city right now, but his stylists are more reasonable.

Oscar Blandi Salon, 746 Madison Ave., 212-988-9404 (haircut with Oscar, $550; with other stylists, $115 and up). If you're stuck in a hair rut, Oscar knows the transformational power of hair—as evidenced by what he did for Reese Witherspoon on Oscar night 2007.

Serge Normant at John Frieda Salon, 825 Washington St. near Little W. 12th St., 212-675-0001; or 30 E. 76th St., 212-879-1000 (cut with Serge, $500; with others, $125). This talented French charmer is constantly zipping around the globe (Elizabeth Hurley's wedding in Mumbai!), so you might have to wait for an appointment for sexy hair if you are not Sarah Jessica Parker or Julia Roberts.

Sally Hershberger Downtown, 425 W. 14th St., Floor 2, 212-206-8700 (cut with Sally, $800; with staff, $100–$250). To get shagged by Sally is something to dine out on. But if you love Meg Ryan's tousled cut or Jane Fonda's modern look, you'll get it for less from her stylists.

Stephen Knoll, 625 Madison Ave., Floor 2, 212-421-0100 (cut with Stephen, $400). He's done a laundry list of celebrities and models for magazine covers.

Blow Styling Salon, 342 W. 14th St. near 9th Ave., 212-989-6282 (blow-out, $40 and up). They don't cut or color, just blow-dry in a cute setting.

Frédéric Fekkai, Henri Bendel, 712 Fifth Ave., Floor 4, 212-753-9500, or 394 W. Broadway, Floor 2, 212-888-2600 (blow-out, $65 and up). For an expert blow-out in midtown, see creative director Mark DeVincenzo or stylist Brandon Shin at this luxurious, 9000-square-foot, state-of-the-art aerie. Downtown, ask for creative director Fabrice Gili, Marshall Lin, or Amanda Malatesta.

Hair Extensions

LaVar Hair Designs (Ellin LaVar), 134 W. 72nd St., 212-724-4492 (extensions, $500–$600). Ellin has her own invisible braid technique for extension perfection, and has amplified the strands of Julia Roberts, Donatella Versace, Naomi Campbell, Whitney Houston, and Mary J. Blige. She's considered the best in the city for African American hair, and her cuts start at $60.

Paul Labrecque Salon, 160 Columbus Ave., 212-988-7816, or 171 E. 65th St., 212-595-0099 (extensions, $2,500–$4,000 for a full head of long hair). After an initial consultation, owner Paul Labrecque orders your color and length from Hairdreams. Another visit, and he attaches this high-quality human hair to small strands of your own. His work is so flawless that people can't tell.

Waxing

Completely Bare, 764 Madison Ave., 212-717-9300 (Basic Bikini, $38; Brazilian, $68; Completely Bare, $75). Three locations in New York City for every kind of waxing, plus laser hair reduction.

J. Sisters International, 35 W. 57th St., 212-750-2485 (Brazilian, $65). The sisters have become synonymous with the Brazilian, their most requested service. Our model Suzy swears by Joyce.

Kimara Ahnert (Lidia Tivichi), 1113 Madison Ave., 212-452-4252 (waxing, $75 and up).

Palm Beach

Facials

Tammy Fender Holistic Skincare, 711 N. Flagler Dr., W. Palm Beach, 561-659-2229 (facials with Tammy, $175; with others, $125 and up). Tammy says, "It is my honor to be part of your journey to be your best self." Love that!

Georgette Klinger Salon (Eiko), 150 Worth Ave., 561-659-1522 (facials, $100–$350).

Nails

George Elliott Salon (Gina), 317 Peruvian Ave., 561-655-3537 (manicure, $25; pedicure, $60; reflexology pedicure, $95). A full-service salon one block north of Worth Avenue.

Annette Vasile, 561-308-4342 (manicure, $30; pedicure, $50). Annette, who prides herself on immaculate tools and natural products, comes to your home, yacht, or hotel room so you can multi-task while you get polished.

Hair

Frédéric Fekkai at the Brazilian Court Hotel (for cuts, Creative Director Bernard Arapoglou or Dris Ramdane), 301 Australian Ave., 561-833-9930 (cuts, $125 and up). This is the premier beauty salon in town, overlooking the pool of an elegant old-world Mediterranean-style hotel that dates back to the Roaring Twenties.

Klinger Advanced Aesthetics (for color, Melissa Peverini), 2511 S. Dixie Hwy., W. Palm Beach, 561-833-1228 (single process, $95; highlights, $200 and up). The sister salon to Georgette Klinger in Palm Beach.

Waxing

Completely Bare Spa, 304 S. County Rd., 561-837-9595 (basic, $38; Brazilian, $68; completely bare, $75). The Palm Beach outpost of this New York hair-removal mecca is where everyone goes for her Brazilian—and more.

Massage

The Spa at The Breakers, 1 S. County Rd., 561-653-6656 (massage, $170 and up). You don't have to be a hotel guest to get pampered at this 140-acre beachfront hotel, resplendent in all its Italian Renaissance–style glory.

Babor Institut Palm Beach (Armi Niemi), 340 Royal Poinciana Plaza, W. Palm Beach, 561-832-9385, babor-institut.com (massage, $95 an hour and up).

Park City, Utah

Brows and Waxing
Alina's Body Retreat, 4677 Nelson Ct., 801-554-2385 (brows, $15 and up; bikini wax, $25 and up). According to writer Bari Nan Cohen, Alina Coleman's salon is the best-kept secret, where every local in the know goes.

Nails
Mountain Body Spa and Cosmetic Deli, 825 Main St., 435-655-9342, mountainbody.com (Salt and Honey spa manicure, $35; pedicure, $45). If you like all-natural skin products, don't leave without perusing the herbal deli of delights, starring salt from the nearby Great Salt Lake.

The Spa at Stein Ericksen Lodge, 7700 Stein Way, Deer Valley, 435-645-6475, steinlodge.com (manicures, $65 in winter, $55 in summer; pedicures, $75 in winter, $65 in summer). This spa offers waxing, too. For head-to-toe pampering, this winter wonderland is the luxe choice.

Hair
Marc Raymond Salon and Spa (Bratis Peralta), Silver Mountain Sports Club, 2080 Gold Dust Ln., 435-649-9680 (haircut, $48 and up; color, $65 and up). A favorite of residents and visiting celebs.

Philadelphia

Brows
Citrus Salon & Day Spa (Michelle), 1201 DeKalb Pike, Blue Bell, 610-277-4247, citrussalonspa.com (brow wax with lesson, $40). Won Best of Philly for Brow Shaping from *Philadelphia* magazine.

Facials
Pierre and Carlo Salon & Spa, Park Hyatt at the Bellevue, 215-790-9910 (Signature Facial, $90).
Rescue Rittenhouse Spa (Danuta Mieloch, owner), 255 S. 17th St., 215-772-2766, rescuerittenhousespa.com (High-Performance Facial, including microdermabrasion, peel, electrocurrent, and oxygen blast, $200). Visit the Web site to take a virtual tour of this great-looking salon, where the staff believes that "beautiful skin is a matter of choice, not chance." They do everything well here, including makeup ($75).

Nails
Ame, 111 Waynewood Ave., Wayne, 610-995-2631 (Sake manicure, $32). A Japanese spa in the 'burbs.
Pierre and Carlo Salon & Spa, Park Hyatt at the Bellevue, 215-790-9910 (pedicure, $50). Excellent pedicure, very relaxing.

Sunless Tanning
Adolf Biecker Spa/Salon, 210 W. Rittenhouse Sq., 215-735-6404 (sunless tanning, $90).
Le Masque, 127 S. State St., Newtown, 215-860-7718 (spray tan, $40). Get airbrushed in Bucks County at aesthetician and makeup artist Johanna Baltes's place. You choose your own shade.

Hair

Richard Nicholas Hair Studio (Erin Porsia), 1716 Sansom St., 215-567-4790 (Dimensional Color, $120).

Studio B (Bart Rosenstein), 58 Fetters Mill Sq., Huntingdon Valley, 215-938-9900. The owner of this cool shop, Bart gives great color, and he knows how to keep a secret.

Head Area @ Matthew Izzo Lifestyle (Lee or JoJo), 1109 Walnut St., 215-829-0699 (haircuts, $45 and up). Everyone buzzes about this boutique's precision cuts . . . and its two-month wait list.

Pileggi on the Square, 717 Walnut St., 215-627-0565 (haircuts, $85 and up; highlights, $110 and up). A busy place with eighteen stylists, housed in a charming five-story town house. The staff cares about the finishing touches, and you walk out feeling like a star, with hair that looks good for days.

Salon 360, 1940 County Line Rd., Huntingdon Valley, 215-953-8100. Big shop, lots of talent.

Waxing

International Salon (Emma Sherby), 1714 Sansom St., 215-563-1141 (bikini, $25; Brazilian, $35). See the amazing Emma for a five-minute Brazilian.

Body Restoration, 1611 Walnut St., 215-569-9599 (half-leg, $35–$40; Brazilian, $60–$75).

San Francisco

Brows

European Skin Care (Lana Kessel), 564 Market St., 415-640-7652 (brows, $35–$40).

Marilyn Jaeger Skincare Studio (Marilyn Jaeger), 415 Spruce St., 415-751-0647 (brows with Marilyn, $39).

Benefit Cosmetics, 2117 Fillmore St., 415-567-0242 (brows, $18–$20). For eyebrow emergencies: Benefit Brow Bars at Macy's and Bloomingdale's (no appointment necessary).

Yelena Spa (Yelena Blumin), 166 Geary St., 415-397-2484 (brow grooming, $35).

Facials

Marilyn Jaeger Skincare Studio (Marilyn Jaeger), 415 Spruce St., 415-751-0647 (facial, $60 and up).

Spa Radiance, 3011 Fillmore St., 415-346-6281 (facial, $115). Sharon Stone and Mary J. Blige have walked through these doors.

Yelena Spa (Yelena Blumin), 166 Geary St., 415-397-2484 (Eminence Facial, $145).

Nob Hill Spa, Huntington Hotel, 1075 California St., 415-345-2888 (facial, $125 and up).

Reméde Spa, St. Regis, 25 Third St., 415-284-4060 (customized facial, $165). The staff also does self-tanning ($130) and antiaging manicures ($55) and pedicures ($65).

Nails

Spa Radiance, 3011 Fillmore St., 415-346-6281 (manicure, $25; pedicure, $45 and up).

Nob Hill Spa, Huntington Hotel, 1075 California St., 415-345-2888 (pedicure, $125 and up).

Elizabeth Arden Red Door Salon & Spa (Faina Golovin), 126 Post St., 415-989-4888 (manicure, $25; pedicure, $48).

Silk Hands & Feet Spa, 1425 Franklin St., 415-885-3277 (manicure, $15).

Sunless Tanning

Brown Sugar Airbrush Tanning Boutique, 1996 Union St., 415-346-3680, brownsugarboutique.net (customized mist-on tanning, $50 and up).

Hair

Joseph Cozza Salon at Gump's, 30 Maiden Lane, Floor 5, 415-433-3030 (single process, $78 and up). Go to Graham Brownlee for terrific color.
Joseph Cozza Salon at the Four Seasons Hotel, 747 Market St., Floor 4, 415-633-3933 (haircut with Sebastien Oxner, $110; color with Angela Berk: single process, $83 and up; highlights, $165 and up). The salon of choice for the cofounders of Benefit Cosmetics, the Ford twins Jean and Jane, which must make it the best in the Bay Area.
77 Maiden Lane Salon & Spa, 77 Maiden Lane, 415-391-7777 (color and highlights, $135 and up). For color, see Christopher Braun or Lisa Nguyen.
DiPietro Todd Salon, multiple locations, dipietrotodd.com (haircut, $250; highlights, $215). Andrew Todd, who works at all locations, will give you a great cut. At 2239 Fillmore St., 415-674-4366, see Emily Kern for color; at 177 Post St., 415-397-0177, see Troy Paine.

Waxing

Marilyn Jaeger Skincare Studio (Marilyn Jaeger), 415 Spruce St., 415-751-0647 (Brazilian waxes, $59 with staff; $63 with Marilyn). Marilyn has been dubbed "the most famous remover of unwanted hair this side of Schick."
The Flying Beauticians, 166 Geary St., Suite 900, 415-391-8929, flyingbeauticians.com (full leg, $85 and up). Mother and daughter European-style esthetician team. Also at 18 East Blithedale, Suite 11, Mill Valley, 415-381-8134.

Seattle

Brows

Red Salon (Angela Bern, owner), 1925 Third Ave., 206-256-6214, redseattle.net (brows with Angela, $35). Angela was the star brow groomer at Christy Carner's until she opened her own hot salon, where she designs brows and more. You may have to wait for an appointment, but she's worth it.
Robert Leonard Salon & Day Spa (June Jaffee), 2033 Sixth Ave., 206-441-9900 (brows, $30). Jaffee is a former hairdresser who has refocused her attention on brows and makeup.

Facials

Ageless Center for Rejuvenation, 601 N. 34th St., Suite C, 206-467-1000, agelessinseattle.com (signature facial, $100). A first-rate medi-spa under the direction of Dr. Barbara Schell, a cosmetic surgeon and dermatologist. A place where savvy Seattleites go for much more than facials.
Red Salon (Angela Bern, owner), 1925 Third Ave., 206-256-6214, redseattle.net (facials, $100 and up). Angela's antiaging facials also give a lot of TLC to the hands, feet, and décolletage, so that they don't tell all. This is a full-service salon that even offers Closet Clean-Up and Wardrobe Consulting.

Nails

Deborah Lippmann Manicure Bar at Nordstrom (Rachelle Adams), 500 Pine St., 206-628-2111 (manicure, $25; pedicure, $45). Deborah Lippmann books up most days, so it's best to make an appointment.
Frenchy's Day Spa, 3131 E. Madison, Suite 103, 206-325-9582 (Frenchy's Manicure, $25; pedicure, $38–$47). Much acclaim for the top-tier Lulu of All Pedicures ($47), which includes scrubbing and buffing with Babor beauty treats.

Sunless Tanning

Cepia Dermotique, 2737 Western Ave. 206-443-0100, cepiadermotique.com (tanning, $25). This chic salon in trendy Belltown has you step into a futuristic skin pod chamber and select your spray from a touch screen offering three shades of tan. You'll be pasty in Seattle no more.

Hair

Gary Manuel Salon (Gary Howse), 2127 First Ave., 206-728-1234, garymanuel.com (cuts with Gary, $160; highlights, $135 and up). When you think of hair salons in Seattle, put this one at the top of the list. And for good reason. Co-owner Gary Howse is known for his multidimensional color as well as his cuts.

Gene Juarez Salon and Spa (Christophe Soltane), eight locations, 206-326-6000, genejuarez.com (cut, $150). If you're new in town or your regular stylist can't take you, go where there are many talented stylists who do amazing, reliably excellent work. Gene Juarez is a good place if you need multiple services (like brow waxing, manicures, and pedicures).

Bocz Salon (Danny Velasquez), 1523 Sixth Ave., 206-624-9134, boczsalon.com (cuts with Danny, $160). Danny Velasquez won *seven* hair accolades from *Seattle* magazine, including Best Overall Stylist and Best Blowout. He knows from fashion-forward hair but doesn't turn off those who want to stay conservative.

Seven (Rodger Azadganian, Amy Troutman), 1520 Seventh Ave. or 101 Bellevue Sq., 206-903-1777, 7salon.com (cuts with Rodger Azadganian, $200; single process, $125; partial highlights, $165). One of Seattle's best cutters, owner Rodger Azadganian believes that the sidewalk is your runway. Color director Amy Troutman gets high praise for her natural-looking shades.

Marco Two Union Square (for cuts, Ric; for color, Walter Jager), 601 Union St., Suite 220, 206-628-8881 (cuts with Ric, $150 and up; single process, $100 and up; partial highlights, $150 and up; full highlights, $175 and up). Sexy with a scissor, Ric has been compared to Warren Beatty in *Shampoo.* Walter Jager is said to really "get" blond.

Waxing

Ummelina Day Spa, 1525 Fourth Ave., 800-663-4SPA (bikini wax, $40). This retreat has an Eastern vibe so you can transport yourself to another world while getting waxed. Owner Nina Ummel also does one of the best pedicures in town (in a private room) for $80.

Habitude at the Locks, 513 N. 36th St., 206-633-1339, or 2801 N.W. Market St., 206-782-2898, habitude.com (waxing, $40–$75). This popular spa has a Northwestern feel and is located within an art gallery with rotating art to keep you entertained. Its mission: "To love and amaze our customers."

Washington, D.C.

Brows and Lashes

Piaf Day Spa & Salon, 1023 15th St. N.W., 202-783-3334 (lash extensions, $350).

Erwin Gomez Salon and Spa, 1519 Wisconsin Ave. N.W., 202-333-7290 (brow grooming with Erwin, $55; follow-up, $40). Erwin, who is said to be the best eyebrow man in town, has a hot new salon in the middle of Georgetown.

Celadon Day Spa (Jacqueline Boucher), 1180 F St. N.W., 202-347-3333 (waxing, $35; tweezing, $38).

Facials

Anabella Spa, 1320 Old Chainbridge Rd., McLean, VA, 703-847-9003 (facials, $80 and up). Washingtonians cross the bridge for "amazing" facials that include a vigorous shoulder massage. Owner Ana Reyes believes in healthy, vibrant, beautiful skin without cosmetic surgery.

Erwin Gomez Salon and Spa, 1519 Wisconsin Ave. N.W., 202-333-7290 (Oxygen-Booster Facial, $180). Catherine Layrle gives a fabulous facial.

Celadon Day Spa (Luci-Eliza Straubel), 1180 F St. N.W., 202-347-3333 (Apple and Paprika Exfoliating Treatment, $110).

Serenity Day Spa, 4000 Wisconsin Ave. N.W., 202-362-2560 (Signature Facial with Micky Keren, $85). Micky gets high grades for being thorough.

Washington Institute of Dermatologic Laser Surgery, 1430 K St. N.W., Floor 2, 202-785-8855 (basic facial, $350). Dr. Tina Alster's Washington Institute of Dermatologic Laser Surgery is where high-profile Washingtonians go to look good on TV. No wonder it's hard to book.

Sugarhouse Day Spa & Salon (Timi Romanka), 111 N. Alfred St., Alexandria, VA, 703-549-9940 (Skin Glowing Facial, $85 and up).

Makeup

Andre Chreky Salon Spa (Rodney Pinion), 1604 K St. N.W., 202-293-9393 (makeup application, $100). Open seven days. "Walk in, float out" is this salon's motto.

George Four Seasons Spa Salon (Carl), 2828 Pennsylvania Ave. N.W., 202-342-1942 (makeup application, $100).

Nails

Circe Salon & Spa, 123 N. Washington St., Alexandria, VA, 703-519-8528 (regular manicure, $26; Hand Relieving Manicure, $50). This Aveda spa has been featured on *Oprah*—need we say more?

Celadon Day Spa (Mina Zihamou), 1180 F St. N.W., 202-347-3333 (manicure, $25; pedicure, $50 and up).

Sunless Tanning

Red Door Salon & Spa, 8075 Leesburg Pike, Vienna, VA, 703-448-8388 (St. Tropez Body Bronzer, $140; St. Tropez Express Body Bronzer, $90).

Hair

Mano (Mistik Halici), 5454 Wisconsin Ave., Chevy Chase, MD, 301-652-0310 (cut, $100; single process, $90; full highlights, $160). Mistik does great highlights, color, and cuts in this salon located in the heart of Chevy Chase.

Andre Chreky Salon Spa, 1604 K St. N.W., 202-293-9393 (single process color, $80; highlights, $120–$150). This full-service salon in a historic town house aims to be a respite of calm for White House staffers and Capitol Hill types. It also gets its share of out-of-towners: Angelina Jolie, Janet Jackson, Salma Hayek, Diane Keaton, Julianne Moore.

O Salon (Dimitri Ferrer), 1079 Wisconsin Ave. N.W., 202-338-9100, osalon.com (half highlights, $130 and up; full highlights, $160 and up).

Okyo Salon (Bernard Portelli, owner), 2903 M St. N.W., 202-342-2675 (base color, $95; highlights, $150 and up). Bernard has built his reputation on color, and even did Catherine Deneuve's. Now he's booked by everyday Washingtonians as well as boldface names. Senator Barbara Boxer, Larry King, John Travolta, and Eva Longoria have all been here. Okyo does hair extensions, too.

Piaf Hair Salon & Day Spa (Lisette Attias), 1023 15th St. N.W., 202-783-3334 (highlights, $85 and up).

Toka (Nuri Yurt), 3251 Prospect St. N.W., 202-333-5133, tokasalon.com (color, $90 and up). DC power brokers get power hair at one of their locations. Jenna and Barbara Bush go to the flagship salon in Georgetown for Nuri's color and cuts. For Mrs. Bush, Nuri makes a house call.

George Four Seasons Spa Salon, 2828 Pennsylvania Ave. N.W., 202-342-1942 (cut, $100; color, $100 and up; highlights, $140 and up). Murat Durak is good with African American hair; Turgay Yavuz has a great eye for color.

Waxing

Bluemercury (Christa Rice), 3059 M St. N.W., 202-965-1300 (full leg wax, $70; bikini wax, $40 and up).

Spa

Nusta Spa, 1129 20th St. N.W., 202-530-5700. An environmentally friendly spa that doesn't skimp on pampering.

The Spa at the Mandarin Oriental, 1330 Maryland Ave. S.W., 202-787-6100. Full-service luxe.

Your Go-To List

Places to Shop

Bare Necessities,
barenecessities.com or
877-728-9272
Barneys New York,
barneys.com
Bath & Body Works,
bathandbodyworks.com or
800-756-5005
Benefit,
benefitcosmetics.com or
800-781-2336
Bigelow Chemists,
bigelowchemists.com or
800-793-5433
Bloomingdale's,
bloomingdales.com or
800-232-1854
Bumble and Bumble,
bumbleandbumble.com or
800-7-BUMBLE
Chanel, chanel.com
Clarins, clarins.com
Clinique, clinique.com
Corinne McCormack,
corinnemccormack.com

Creative Nail Design,
creativenaildesign.com
Dermalogica,
dermalogica.com
Essie Cosmetics, essie.com
Estée Lauder,
esteelauder.com
Everything But Water,
everythingbutwater.com
Farouk Systems, farouk.com
or 800-237-9175
Figleaves, figleaves.com
Fresh, fresh.com or
800-FRESH-20
HairDo, hsn.com
Hairdreams, hairdreams.com
HairMax, hairmaxshop.com
or 866-527-3726
Hanes, onehanesplace.com
or 800-671-1674
Hanky Panky, hankypanky
.com or 212-725-4996
Her Room, herroom.com or
800-558-6779
Insolia, insolia.com
Kevyn Aucoin,
kevynaucoin.com
Kiehl's, kiehls.com
La Mer, lamer.com
Lancôme Paris,
lancome.com
Laura Mercier,
lauramercier.com
LensCrafters,
lenscrafters.com
Lipo in a Box,
lipoinabox.com

Lippmann Collection,
lippmanncollection.com
MAC Cosmetics,
maccosmetics.com or
800-588-0070
Macy's, macys.com or
800-289-6229
Maidenform,
maidenform.com
Mark, meetmark.com
NARS, narscosmetics.com
Neiman Marcus,
whatshebuys.com or
888-888-4757
NIOXIN, nioxin.com or
800-628-9890
Nordstrom, nordstrom.com
or 888-282-6060
Norva Barber Supply,
norvabarbersupply.com or
800-542-0111
NYCE Legs, nycelegs.com or
866-692-3534
OPI, opi.com
Parissa, parissa.com or
888-986-9974
philosophy, philosophy.com
Prescriptives,
prescriptives.com
Robert Marc Boutiques,
212-675-5200 for locations or
robertmarc.com
Rogaine, rogainedirect.com
or 888-835-9712

Scott Barnes,
scottbarnes.com
Senna Cosmetics,
sennacosmetics.com
Sephora, sephora.com or
877-SEPHORA
Shu Uemura,
shuuemura-usa.com or
888-SHU-5678
Skin Store, skinstore.com
Smashbox, smashbox.com
Spanx, spanx.com or
800-806-7311
Speedo, the-swim-store.com
Target, target.com
Tracie Martyn,
traciemartyn.com
Tweezerman, tweezerman
.com or 800-645-3340
Victoria's Secret,
victoriassecret.com or
800-411-5116
Wolford, wolford.com or
800-WOLFORD

Experts to Call

Chris Cusano, hairstylist
Red Door Spa at Elizabeth
Arden
691 Fifth Ave.
New York, NY 10022
212-546-0200
Dr. Gervaise Gerstner,
dermatologist
Park Avenue Skin Care
1130 Park Ave.

New York, NY 10128
212-369-9600
Dr. Jeff Golub-Evans,
cosmetic dentist
New York Center for Cosmetic
Dentistry
128 East 71st St.
New York, NY 10021
212-288-4455
Dr. Melanie Grossman,
dermatologist
161 Madison Ave.
New York, NY 10016
212-725-8600
Antoinette Guzzo, hairstylist
antoinetteguzzo@mac.com or
646-732-1421
Dr. James Jacobs, D.M.D.,
periodontist
30 Central Park South
New York, NY 10019
212-371-5250
Brad Johns, colorist
Global Color Director, Clairol
National Color Director, Red
Door Spa at Elizabeth Arden
691 Fifth Ave.
New York, NY 10022
212-546-0200

Ellin LaVar, hairstylist
LaVar Hair Designs
134 West 72nd St.
New York, NY 10023
212-724-4492
info@lavarhairdesigns.com
Donna Lennon, bra specialist
Drawer Full of Lingerie
2200 Glades Rd.
Boca Raton, FL 33431
561-394-2424
Terri Levin, laser specialist
Laser Hair Removal for Men
and Women
631-588-1100
laserhairremovalformenand
women.com
Dr. Suzanne Levine,
podiatrist
885 Park Ave.
New York, NY 10021
212-535-0229
Dr. Martin Polin, cosmetic
dentist
2600 Military Trail, Suite 320
Boca Raton, FL 33431
561-997-2323
Dr. Neil Sadick,
dermatologist
Sadick Dermatology Center
911 Park Ave.
New York, NY 10021
212-772-7242
Dr. Robert Schwartz,
cosmetic dentist
220 Central Park South,
Suite 1A
New York, NY 10019
212-541-9500

213

Sharyn Soleimani, personal shopper
Barneys New York
660 Madison Ave.
New York, NY 10021
212-833-2606

Susan Sommers, fashion coach
DressZing
411 West End Ave.
New York, NY 10024
212-877-4963
dresszing.com

Joseph Ting, tailor
Dynasty Tailors
6 East 38th St.
New York, NY 10016
212-679-1075

Dr. Patricia Wexler, dermatologist
145 East 32nd St.
New York, NY 10016
888-WEXLER-MD
patriciawexlermd.com

Robert Sweet William,
The Brow Man
Barneys New York
660 Madison Ave.
New York, NY 10021
212-833-2606

Dr. Allan Wulc, dermatologist
847 Easton Rd., Suite 1500
Warrington, PA 18976
215-918-5552

Resources Referred to in This Book

WEB SITES

American Academy of Cosmetic Surgery, cosmeticsurgery.org
American Society of Laser Medicine Surgery, aslms.org
Bottomless Closet, bottomlesscloset.org
Clairol, clairolusa.com
Dress for Success, dressforsuccess.org
Lion's Clubs, lionsclubs.org
Society of Permanent Cosmetic Professionals, spcp.org
Vision Council of America, vca.com
Weight Watchers, weightwatchers.com
Cotton Inc., cottoninc.com

BOOKS

Beauty Junkies
by Alex Kuczynski
I Feel Bad About My Neck
by Nora Ephron
Inventing the Rest of Our Lives
by Suzanne Braun Levine
Leap! by Sara Davidson
The Power Years
by Ken Dychtwald
and Daniel J. Kadlec

Credits

The "Size Matters" chart in chapter 13, page 125, originally appeared in *Shop, Etc.,* a publication of Hearst Communications, Inc.

Thank-Yous

Truth be told . . . this book would never have happened if Judy Linden of the Stonesong Press didn't call me out of the blue for lunch one day when I was executive editor at *Shop Etc.* magazine. She had just seen my *Today* show segment about jeans and thought the time was right for a book about them. After we tossed around the idea a bit, it become clear to me that I was interested in only one aspect of jeans: how wearing the right pair can make you look ten years younger! I got excited about all the things you can do to shave off the years, and I presented the list to Judy. For all I knew (we didn't know each other that well), she would just continue her search for someone dying to write about jeans. I'm forever grateful that she didn't. From that day forward, Judy became the first and most passionate believer in *How Not to Look Old.* She is my partner on this book, and I could never have done it without her.

Shopping this book . . . was a little like going through sorority rush. A dozen publishers tried to convince us that they were *the* house. We could not have found a better home than the Springboard imprint of Grand Central Publishing. My deepest gratitude to the extraordinary Karen Murgolo, who had the vision to propel this into a "focus" book and then the guts to take giant steps out of the box to assure that it didn't look and feel like every other style guide. Heartfelt thanks to Jamie Raab, who "got it" from the start and so enthusiastically championed this project that she let it be known that this was the only proposal she has ever kept in her desk drawer "for quick reference."

Special thanks to classy Matthew Ballast for getting the word out so expertly and creatively.

And thanks to the believers at Hachette Book Group USA who made it all happen: Suzanne Albert, Emi Battaglia, Melissa Bullock, Peggy Freudenthal, Tom Hardej, Jayne Yaffe Kemp, Julia Kushnirsky, Diane Luger, Anne Twomey, Pam Schechter.

My backup team . . . was the terrific Stonesong Press. I so appreciate the unwavering support and enormous contributions of Ellen Scordato, Alison Fargis, Paul Fargis, and Oriana Leckert. For original research, reporting, and fact-checking, I depended on a small group of loyal and dedicated young journalists. Big thanks to the remarkable Brette Polin for always being there for me from the very beginning. Special thanks to Ayren Jackson-Cannady for sharing her expertise. Thanks to Tanvi Chheda for her skillful fact-checking and to Kate Gleason for research.

I so appreciate the words of three gifted writers. Heartfelt thanks to Sally Wadyka, who saved the day with her speedy, lively prose. To Michele Orecklin for her all her eloquent wordplay. To Melissa Schweiger, the original Y&H woman, for her way with fashion.

The look of the book . . . is thanks to the visionary Cicero DeGuzman, Jr., a creative genius whose powerful pages incorporated all the many moving parts without sacrificing elegance, sophistication, beauty, and clarity. His dynamic and dramatically different design transcends the expected. I'm honored to have been Cicero's first book (which won't be his last!).

The glam quotient . . . ramped up with rocket fuel the minute the beauty and fashion photographer Timothy Hogan signed on for all the original photography. His discerning eye and lavish lighting make everything and everyone look maximally gorgeous. Thanks to Timothy and his team for three days of photographic bliss. And to our tireless photography wrangler, Agatha Wasilewska, for securing the photographic A-team and for poring over thousands of celebrity photos in search of age appropriateness. Much appreciation for the perfecting talents of our first-rate glam squad—makeup artist Jenna Anton and hairstylist Amy Farid. I can never say thank you enough to the Genevieve Yraola, the style queen, whose dedication, imagination, and cool permeated every photo and fashion chapter. She has styled many of my best TV segments, and I don't know how I'd live without her! Thanks to Kimmi Ade, who expertly assisted.

Finding three models over forty who everyone could relate

to . . . was not easy. At the end of two fruitless days of model casting, I turned to my friend since high school, the effervescent and multitalented Laurette Kittle, who lives in Greenwich, Connecticut, and knows everyone. I can't thank her enough for enthusiastically sending our way three of her friends, Michelle Hesse, Jillian Aufderheide, and Suzy Marek Armstrong, all fabulous can-do women whose optimism and high energy made the Y&H concepts come alive.

For the proposal . . . this project got liftoff thanks to the early love, support, and magical creativity of the smart marketing duo of Della Olsher and Erica Levine. I'm so grateful for the friendship of the brilliant creative director Nora Sheehan, who shared her fresh artistic direction. An enormous thank-you to the photographer Keith Lathrop for generously allowing me to use the head shot he took of me, on the cover of the blad.

For the cover . . . A big kiss to photographer Michael Waring for making me look taller and thinner than I deserve to. . . . And to Julie Harris (and Timothy Priano) for makeup . . . and to Corey Morris for hair.

The experts . . . are the heart of this book. Almost every single person whose time and expertise I asked for responded with an enthusiastic "Happy to help!" I so appreciate the hours they spent talking with me and responding to follow-up e-mails with no-spin honesty. Many of my experts are cherished members of my personal beauty and fashion A-team. They make me look young day in, day out. I definitely couldn't have done this book without . . .

Efrat Acharkam
Nick Barose
Sara Blakely
Dr. Mitch Cassel
Chris Cusano
Yves de Chiris
Gervaise Gerstner, M.D.
Jeff Golub-Evans, D.D.S.
R. J. Graziano
Melanie Grossman, M.D.
Antoinette Guzzo
Liz Hosofar
James Jacobs, D.M.D.
Brad Johns
Lois Joy Johnson
Neil Lane
Ellin LaVar
Donna Lennon
Terri Levin

Suzanne Levine, D.P.M.
Deborah Lippmann
Robert Marc
Corinne McCormack
Isaac Mizrahi
Martin R. Polin, D.M.D.
Neil Sadick, M.D.
Robert Schwartz, D.M.D.
Sharyn Soleimani
Susan Sommers
Susan Sterling
Joseph Ting
Patricia Wexler, M.D.
Robert Sweet William
Alan Wulc, M.D., F.A.C.S.
Genevieve Yraola

To friends in the biz . . . who went way above and beyond helping me to get every single detail right. My love and thanks to the gorgeous Lois Joy Johnson for her extraordinary generosity, friendship, and willingness to share every name, every product, everything she knows about fashion and beauty (which is a lot!). The brilliant Brad Johns for having an expert take on everything and the patience to share it all with me. The amazing Gloria Appel, who, along with Larry Appel, shared her collective savvy in the marketing department. The visionary Lisa Gabor for her expert and strategic editing. The irrepressible Jane Berk for reading and tweaking every chapter. The product queen Julie Redfern for shopping with me at Sephora. The refreshing Gervaise Gerstner, who makes it a joy to see the doctor.

To Cindy Lewis, Barbara Graustark, Kim Isaacsohn, Lisa Glinsky, Lora Nasby, and Terry Krupp, who tested beauty by the bagfuls.

To Anne Keating, Cynthia Parsons, Janet Gurwitch, Camille McDonald, and Mary Mayotte for all their brilliant big ideas.

To Mindy Grossman for her passionate support of this project at HSN.

And someone I can never thank enough is the fearless Katie Couric, who, in over a decade of friendship, has always been there for me with smart advice and inspiration and whose early support of the book meant so much.

The _Today_ show staff . . . produced more than 130 amazing segments on style for me over the past ten years, many of which are mentioned in these pages. I owe the hosts and producers past and present big-time for their professionalism and continued support: Jim Bell, Amy Rosenblum, Marc Victor, Jonathan Wald, Tom Touchet, Linda Finnell, Betsy Alexander, Katie Couric, Matt Lauer, Natalie Morales, Ann Curry, Al Roker, Margaret Pergler, Rainy Farrell, Cecelia Fang, Cheryl Wells . . . and I don't know how I can ever truly thank the incomparable Jeff Zucker for putting me on _Today_ way back in January 1996 and for his friendship and loyalty through my many magazine-editor incarnations.

The _Oprah_ staff . . . produced many groundbreaking segments mentioned in this book. Special thanks for the generous support of Oprah Winfrey, Lisa Erspamer, Jill Barancik, and Rita Thompson.

The _Shop Etc._ staff . . . continued to be caring and supportive friends well after the magazine folded. Heartfelt thanks to my talented former colleagues Karen Catchpole, Kate Dimmock, Clio McNichol, Charles Short, Sara Sugarman, Andrea Rosengarten, and Paula Tushbai. And big thanks to Wendy Israel at Hearst for granting permission to reprint from _Shop Etc._

To my friends in the fashion and beauty biz . . . a round of thanks for loaning us clothes, accessories, shoes, shapewear, and beauty products:

Alison Brod, Rayna Greenberg, and Carly Abel at Alison Brod
Nancy Behrman, Rachel Kane, Lauren Rodolitz, Laura Bierbaum, and Simona Levin at Behrman

Anne Keating, Kelly Moro McKay, and Elizabeth Quarta at Bloomingdale's
Laura Wright and Kristen Marturano, formerly at Blue Sky
Tara Madden and Meg Robinson at Bratskeir & Co.
Nicole Matusow at Clarins
Francine Gingras, Helene Leslie, and Brent Miller at Clairol
Erin McCaffrey at Clinique
Merideth Fanning Gilmor and Vanessa LeBlanc at Cole Haan
Samantha Dark
Stephanie Smirnov, Deborah Nadler, Margee Macdonell, and Thea DiChiara Zagata at DeVries
Terri Barnes at Hanes Brands
Lizzie Neary at Donna Karan Intimates
Marianne Diorio and Amy Karches at Estée Lauder
Candance Greever and Bridget Quinn Strickline at Everything but Water
Beth Klein and Denise Davila at Frédéric Fekkai
Kelly McNamara and Veronica Dunn at Giorgio Armani Cosmetics
Shirley Giovetti
Julia Sloan at Guerlain Paris
Robert Heim at HairDreams
Korey Provencher at Isaac Mizrahi
Mark Marinovich and Jan Marini at Jan Marini
Corinne Zadigan at Jo Malone
Joanne Chiu and Rachael Kelley at Kiehl's
Leslie Stevens and Simone Delfino at LaForce & Stevens
Kerry Diamond at Lancôme

Michael Trese, Franca Gerrard, Blair Crames, and Arlene Benza at L'Oréal Paris
Connie Elder of Lipo-in-a-Box
Maureen Lippe and Lauren Glicken at Lippe Taylor
Marina Maher, Nancy Lowman LaBadie, Lori Dunn, and Jackie Widrow at Marina Maher
Cody Adams and Lindsay Burns at M. Booth
Corinne McCormack
Bruno Zerdoun at Murval
Stacy Gulisano and Jenna Muller at Phyto
Ginger Tiong at Prescriptives
Wendy Converse at R. J. Graziano
Anna Natsume at Robert Marc
Laura Lee at Scott Barnes
Jodi Sandler at Sequin
Harris Shepard
Heidi Manheimer, Jadzia Tirsch, and Nicole Cardillo at Shiseido
Stephanie Boccuzza and Andrea Halpern at Shop PR
Franny Viola, Amanda Smeal, Kerri Ross, and Katie Stratakis at Siren
Kelly Sierra at Tevrow + Chase
Wendy Somes
Misty Elliott and Wendy Lewis at Spanx
Marius Morariu at Tracie Martyn
Erin Laird at Tracy Paul
Tory Burch, Susie Draper, and Kerry Carrera at Tory Burch
Trisha White
Jackie Tractenberg, Jackie Sands, Katie Welch, Kate Hall, and Rebecca Levy at Tractenberg & Co.
Rosemarie Sterling and Rosemary Rodriguez at YSL Beauté

Special thanks for their generous sharing of info: Beth Boyle of NPD, Robin Merlo of Cotton Inc., and Susan Welch at the Vision Council of America.

Brilliant magazine editors . . . I've worked with throughout my career have inspired me. Thank you to Karen Anderegg, Barbara Coffey, Judith Coyne, Bonnie Fuller, Amy Gross, Lois Joy Johnson, Charla Lawhon, Edith Raymond Locke, Martha Nelson, Peggy Northrop, and Mandi Norwood.

To my personal support team . . . thanks for your care and excellent counsel. I'm so happy to have Heidi Krupp, Christianna Capra, Jaime Wolf, and Adam Leibner in my life.

To my family . . . for putting up with me! Thanks to Jay, Lisa, Mollie, and Jami Krupp and to Janet, Larry, Paul, and Rose Zoglin, who totally got the fact that Richard and I just didn't have the time, as we were both writing books for two years!

And heartfelt thanks . . . to you, dear reader, for having the guts to grow and change.

It took a country . . . to produce the twenty-one city lists. I couldn't book that many beauty services personally, so I had to rely on my own Style Network. Big thanks to Steve Boulliane, Jill Brooke, Kim Isaacsohn, Laurette Kittle, Cindy Lewis, Mary Mayotte, Steve and Linda Permut, Susan Sommers, and David Stansbury, as well as other friends and family who graciously introduced me to their beauty-maven friends.

Salons go in and out of style as fast as restaurants, and no one knows that better than Judy Linden, Ellen Scordato, Alison Fargis, and Oriana Leckert. My deepest gratitude for their tireless dedication to fact-checking the names of the beauty pros we listed.

I am forever grateful to the network of beauty mavens willing to share the names and numbers of the best beauty pros in their city without a worry that they may never squeeze in an appointment again! These lists are mostly the subjective opinions of the following people, who helped me sleuth out what salons were still hip (but not too hip). I thank them so much for their generous sharing of the wealth.

Aspen: Lynn Buoniconti, Lily Garfield, Maury Rogoff
Atlanta: Misty Elliott, Wendy Lewis, the women of Spanx, Lisa Tush
Boston: Wendy Pierce, Kate Weinstein
Chicago: Wendy Donahue, Bonnie Kaplan, Terry Krupp, Lynne Meyer, Molly Dava Levy, Jessica Mumaw, Marilu Roffee, Courtney Weinberg, Lila Weinberg
Dallas: Joanne Teichman for her list, Jean Ingersoll, Tracy Hayes
Denver: Donna Crafton, Lesley Kennedy, Mary Mayotte
Detroit: Nicole Avery, Jackie Bean, Beckie Thompson
Houston: Janet Gurwitch and Sharon Collier for their list

Kansas City: Andrea Price, Carol Price, Deborah Shouse, Jackie White, Rose Zoglin

Las Vegas: Angela Rich (who has her manicured finger on the pulse of this town) for her list

Los Angeles: Angela Rich for her list, Cameron Brunner, Ronni Chasen, Brad Johns, Deborah Ramo, Tracey Ross

Miami: Tammi Fuller, Jonny Levy

Minneapolis: Leslie Jablonski, Allison Kaplan

Nashville: Linda Roberts, Connie Elder, Hollie Deese

New York City: Jenna Anton, Jane Berk, Marianne Dougherty, Amy Farid, Lisa Gabor, Antoinette Guzzo, Brad Johns, Lois Joy Johnson, Cindy Lewis, Julie Redfern, Maury Rogoff, Susan Sommers, Dana Wood

Palm Beach: Karen Golov and Suzanne Frank for their lists, Maury Rogoff

Park City, Utah: Bari Nan Cohen for her list (the day after she gave birth!)

Philadelphia: Gigi Wolk

San Francisco: Alison Haljun, Andrea Price, Yetunde Schuhmann, Anne Zehren

Seattle: Audrey Beaulac, Nicole Mertes, Meredeth McMahon, Joanne Plank

Washington, D.C.: Vaneeda Bennett, Trish Malloch Brown, Soraya Chemaly, Erika Kelton, Mandy Locke, Maria Price, Claire Shipman, Cynthia Steele, Caroline Stevens

Meet Our Models:

Michelle, Suzy, and Jillian—all moms, all over forty.

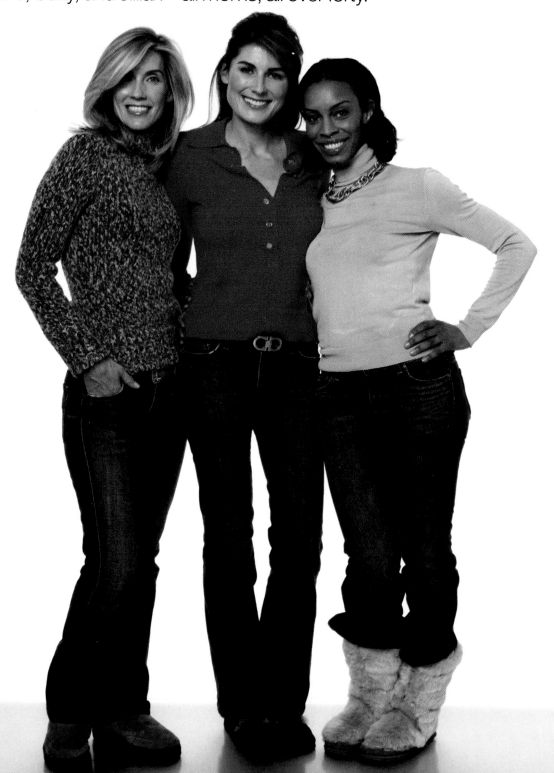